MW01502792

CONTENTS

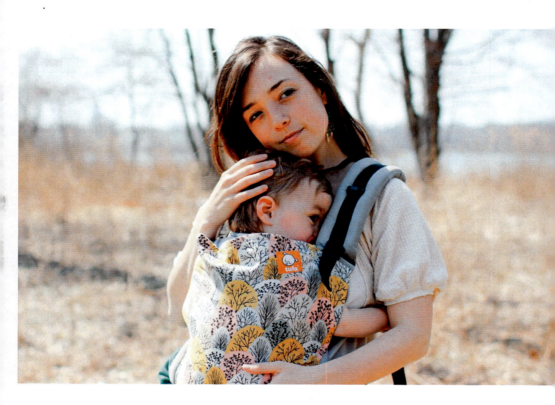

I'm Hadas, a holistic health coach, doula, Pilates instructor, Columbia University alumna, writer, polyglot, photographer, tree-hugger, mother, wife, sister, and daughter. I believe that in order to become our greatest versions, we must remember ourselves as children of Earth and siblings to all, sharing this beautiful and abundant planet. It's my mission to help you connect with Earth's medicines by eating in alignment with her cycles and seasons and by understanding the human body as a microcosm of the Universe. When we learn to eat intuitively and with reverence to the ancient ways, we open ourselves up to a wider and higher perspective that enables us to truly step into our unique magic, to let our paths unfold gracefully, naturally, and in symbiotic relationship with all beings.

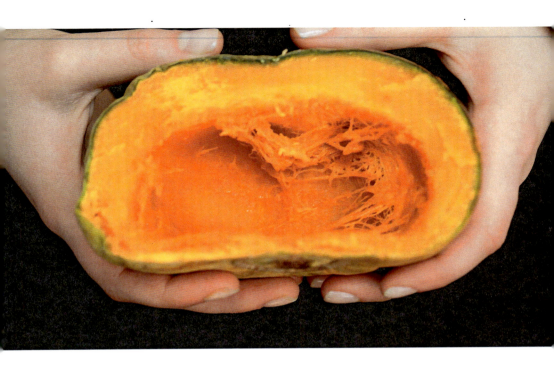

WELCOME, WILD ONE

I'm so grateful to have you here with me on this journey toward higher Self, radiant health, and home-cooking fueled with love and intention. I believe that taking this first step will be nourishing for us both, because when each one of us taps into our greatest version, the benefits ripple out and inspire others to reclaim their *own* health and wisdom.

Let's begin by taking a look at Western medicine versus Eastern medicine, and why I choose a holistic, integrative approach toward healing.

Western medicine does a very good job of suppressing symptoms. If we tell our doctor we feel depressed, they will prescribe us an antidepressant, it will flood our brain with neurotransmitters, and we might begin to feel better. Then we can either continue to take the medication for the rest of our lives, or we can use it to get to a place where we can better help ourselves.

Sometimes the answers slip away from us; internal or external factors (or both!) become too overwhelming to process, and we seek help outside ourselves. There's nothing wrong with asking for help. Sometimes that is the most growth-inspiring and humbling decision we can make in our current state. The issue is that when we wholly rely on pharmaceuticals to heal us, we relinquish all of our power. We don't actually grow from our challenges but become less present in our reality. We think we need a doctor, a pill, an appointment, and a pharmacy to fix us. We haven't found any other way out.

But the ability to heal ourselves is our birthright. We are living in a tiny percentage of human history in which we have lost our connection to Earth, to the Elements, plants, and foods that heal, that guide us deep within so we can shine without.

That memory is still there. We still own it within the ancestral DNA of our bodies, and the tools in this book are here to help you reconnect and reclaim.

As a holistic health practitioner, I don't view depression as a condition that calls for suppression. To the contrary, it calls for deconstruction. In the West, we seem to view disease as a foreign, ambiguous invader which, for no understandable reason, chooses us.

I'm certainly not anti-science, but I do believe that science leaves out a fundamental component of the whole truth: that which we cannot see or measure. My practice specializes in Eastern nutritional medicine, which holds the principle that disease invades the body over time. Even-

tually, if left untreated, it settles in. The emotions involved in depression and anxiety are not isolated emotions that call for suppression medicine. They're actually rooted in our internal organs and ninety percent the results of our diet and lifestyle. For a balanced emotional life, we need to work with our organs and our choices in order to figure out what's really behind the symptoms. We need to look at what spiritual and emotional toxins are invading, in addition to the detectable chemical imbalances.

When we're stuck in a place of darkness and hopelessness, it makes perfect sense why we'd turn to a quick fix. That's what I did when I was depressed some years ago. What I didn't realize is that conventional antidepressants are not really a fix at all. They're Band-aids. With this book, I intend to show another option, and it's rooted in diet and lifestyle.

Ironically, this feels like the most difficult and invasive kind of healing for many of us. We seem to find changing the contents of our refrigerators or restructuring our days more invasive than surgery and other procedures that "restore" our health. We get defensive when someone tells us to give up cheese, but we find it perfectly normal to fix a problem by checking into a hospital, getting undressed, strapped to a table, drugged to sleep, and taking a knife to the insides of our bodies.

We ignore the warning signs our bodies give us until it's too late. But we can learn to heed them, instead. Deep healing through food is often a slow fix, which should be proof enough that it's the first way to go. A problem that takes time to form, takes time to dissolve. When we slow down, we let nature run her course. We can actually download and digest her wisdom. The side effects include self love, greater connection to ourselves, the planet, each other, and the foundation we need to discover and then shine our own, completely unique light.

We might argue that eating healthy food is:

A. Too expensive.

• But aren't antacids, toilet paper, pain relievers, and all the drugs we take to mask our suffering also expensive? Aren't all the beauty products we buy to hide breakouts on our skin also expensive? Skin is, after all, the largest organ in the body and releases toxins through blemishes. Instead of asking why organic food is so expensive, why not ask why GMO and pesticide-grown food is so cheap.

B. We don't have time to grocery shop and cook.

• We have time, though, to wait in the emergency room and to go through surgeries that wipe us out for days, weeks, or longer. We have time to wait on line at the pharmacy for our prescriptions. We have time to sit on the toilet or sleep off the effects of medications. Medicine shouldn't have any side effects. It should just make us feel better. But the medicine we're prescribed can create more side effects than benefits. There's really no such thing as a side effect, anyway. Whatever a medicine causes *is* its effect, period. So when we watch a commercial for an antidepressant, or any drug for that matter, we notice that there are about fifteen seconds of advertising on how great we'll feel on the drug, walking our dog and kissing our spouse of fifty years on the beach, followed by two minutes of how we may also experience heart failure, kidney failure, weight-gain, increased suicidal thoughts...you get the picture.

When we start to shift our perspective, all that's left in making a change is knowing what foods will heal us in all our uniqueness, and how to cook them. That's where this book comes in. Once upon a time our food was medicinal. Now we have medicine without food and food that is void of medicine. We are here to put the medicine back into the food.

Don't worry; the food I recommend is easy to prepare and of course delicious. Nature gifts us with an incredible bounty of colors, flavors, textures, and nutrients. The least we can do is prepare them deliciously, in return! The food we're making is free of additives, preservatives, dyes, pesticides, fertilizers, chemicals, flavorings, artificial sweeteners, and low-quality fats that pervade the food so many of us are accustomed to eating.

Over 6,000 legal chemicals have been allowed in our food chain since WWII. The body doesn't recognize any of these chemicals and views them as foreign invaders. How does the body react to these chemicals? Inflammation. Illness. Disease and *dis-ease*.

You'll notice that I don't push cutting out entire food groups. Though I choose not to eat from certain groups, we should, theoretically, be able to eat everything without experiencing inflammation. The main issue in our food system that is linked to depression and anxiety is the quality and quantity of what we eat.

Even if we avoid GMOs and processed food, it's next to impossible to create a completely organic world for ourselves while living in society. But we can do better.

I will give you the information and tips you need in order to use simple, affordable foods as staples in your diet. I'll explain how to strengthen your digestion so that a little bit of junk food here and there won't harm you. If you can begin to incorporate these tools into your lifestyle, things will shift for you.

This is not to say that everything you've been feeling, that all of the negative thoughts, doubts, or barriers in your life are the result of your diet. In fact, we would all do ourselves a big favor by honoring the fact that our external environment affects our internal environment, too.

Often in the spiritual community, I hear people say "our thoughts create our reality." Yes, this is true. Intention and positive thinking are incredibly powerful tools. But when taken as doctrine or law, we can feel as though our suffering is entirely our fault, that it is a lack on our part that inhibits our healing. But life *happens* just as we *create* life. If we want to free ourselves from suffering, we shouldn't *bypass* uncomfortable emotions. We should actually honor them. We should allow them time to rise to the surface and allow our*selves* times to process them.

When we acknowledge the external environment, we create more space in our minds and clarity in our bodies to listen to what our internal environment is telling us. By honoring our internal environment through nutrient-dense nourishment, we will, at the very least, take the edge off of our suffering. And more likely, it will also bring gifts of clarity, levity, and pleasure on a biochemical level. It is the basis for good health.

Know that just by reading this book, you've already taken the first step on this new path toward healing. You have said "Yes!" to a cascade of vibrancy, health, and intuition. You have signaled to the Universe that you are ready, so get ready!

As I've said, I sought the "normal" way out of depression when I was younger, but once I realized how shallow my healing had really been, I decided to choose a different path by following my gut (pun intended!). I quit my uninspiring office job and worked as a chef for a few years, learning new cooking techniques and making friends with food, with which I was previously in a complicated relationship. I continued my studies as a doula and Pilates instructor as well as a holistic health counselor, which gave me the knowledge that forms the backbone of this book.

During my training, I studied traditional Chinese medicine, Ayurveda, Western and modern scientific research, and cultures of longevity as researched by the Weston A. Price Foundation. Weston Price was a dentist who travelled around the world visiting and researching cultures with particularly long life spans. He discovered that isolated, non-industrialized cultures that stuck to a traditional diet based on the foods available to them had virtually no health issues. As soon as these people left their homes and discovered processed foods, their health completely deteriorated to the point where their jaw structures changed.

My education combined these four ways of looking at food to form a holistic idea of how to eat for longevity, rejuvenation, and healing.

Discovering how a change of diet could affect me so completely, to my very core, made me realize that as I continue to live a life aligned with my values, I have the duty to share what I had the privilege to learn.

This book isn't only for those suffering from depression, anxiety, or mental illness; it's really for anyone who feels ready to elevate their diet and their life. Keep in mind that every time I recommend a food, I'm talking about that food in its highest quality — organic and as local as possible. Though each recipe in this book is vegan, I do refer to animal products for those who choose to consume them, and these should always be pasture-raised or wild animals that were fed their natural diet.

We're going to cover a lot of ground. You won't need any special kitchen equipment (a blender is as wild as it gets); you won't need to travel far for ingredients; you won't need to take out any bank loans; and you'll have plenty of room to add your own unique style and tastes to each and every dish. Now let the healing begin...

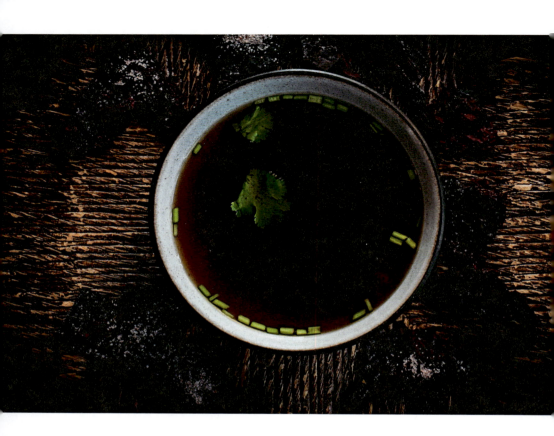

1

IT ALL STARTS WITH DIGESTION

Most of my clients have come to me wanting to lose weight, improve their skin, or deal with a chronic health issue. Yet time and time again, we find that they're really dealing with deeper emotional issues. They tell me they feel anxious, depressed, or can't think clearly. They're always tired. They lack drive, maybe even sex drive. This does not come out immediately for a few reasons, but the one I want to focus on is this: we are so accustomed to thinking these feelings are normal parts of the human condition. In one sense, they are. Life presents challenges. But the kind of chronic fogginess, fatigue, and anxiety that most people deal with on a day-to-day basis is not normal and not something we must simply "learn to live with."

How Digestion Fails

Doctors prescribe us medicine that gives relief as quickly as possible, but it does not address any of our underlying issues or the synergistic way the body works. For example, we take antacids for heartburn. Antacids stop the formation of acid in the stomach; seems great, right? Not exactly. Stomach acid is *necessary* for the digestion of protein. When we don't properly digest our protein, amino acids are not made, which means neurotransmitters are not made. That's when we start to feel depressed and turn to stimulants to improve our mood.

Furthermore, the protein that is not properly digested can begin to ferment, causing the stomach acid to reappear. Over time, drugs like antacids stop working because they completely disable the digestive system. Instead of taking them, we should be addressing the root causes of heartburn, which are coffee, alcohol, smoking, sleeping on a full stomach, overeating, and an overly acidic diet. Then, we can treat people with foods that replace lost stomach acid in an extremely nourishing way (such as umeboshi vinegar, raw apple cider vinegar, lemon) and look to natural foods like aloe vera juice

to relieve acid reflux immediately. Of course, pharmaceutical companies can't profit from fresh aloe vera juice, so its healing properties are less widely advertised. But fixing stomach acid is one example of a way to improve our digestion and, consequently, our mood. Without neurotransmitters like serotonin and dopamine, depression creeps in.

Our digestive system needs to do what it is meant to do. When we inhibit parts of it with drugs, when we subscribe to this over-the-counter way of life, we're creating long-term damage. We shouldn't be blocking acid but resetting our digestive systems altogether!

A person with digestive issues is likely to feel symptoms of spaciness, depression, or lack of focus. Most doctors don't connect the two, but now, researchers are starting to discover how our digestion plays a huge role in our mental health.

The number one way to boost our digestion and improve our mood is through probiotics. Probiotics are microscopic bacterial organisms that promote life. They are the product of fermentation of yeast and sugar. The small and large intestine contain over 100 trillion bacteria. 95% of our body is made up of bacteria. Fermentation is a wild process, making the consumption of fermented foods a way to assimilate the wild into the body. Chinese medicine is all about becoming a part of the natural world through holistic healing, eating with the seasons, eating locally, and following a traditional diet. Consuming the unmediated life force within probiotics helps us adapt to our own changing surroundings. Through consuming fermented foods, we become less susceptible to devastating conditions like depression. We simply connect with ancestral practices of making food digestible, flavorful, and unique.

This last quality, "uniqueness," strikes me as especially topical, as more and more of our food is being genetically modified to grow identically. Every conventional apple has become the same tasteless, waxy, and shiny hybrid, rather than an individual result of the nutrients it absorbed from its soil and relation to the rest of the apples on its tree. When we feel stuck, unmotivated, bland, and depressed, accepting the opposite kind of energy can be just the medicine we need.

Our food was the perfect source of this energy for our ancestors. Let's take a quick look at how vegetables absorb nutrients. The root of a carrot, for example, should be covered in villi that absorb nutrients, microflora, bacteria, fungus, and minerals from the soil. Today, because of widespread pesticide use, the villi of our vegetables as well as our soil have been destroyed. We're left with produce that doesn't nutritionally satisfy us as it once did, and our digestive systems are not nourished as they once were. We used to get probiotics from well water, too, which is, of course, no longer available to most of us.

In our culture, we've completely lost probiotics as a dietary staple. The good bacteria in our gut is further wiped out by antibiotics, birth control, acne medications, and many other pharmaceuticals. Nobody seems to tell us that if we take these drugs, we need to be taking probiotics, as well.

Antibiotics kill good bacteria along with the bad. When that good bacteria is cleared out, yeast in the digestive tract gets free rein. Many women get pregnant completely unaware of how much yeast is in their digestive tract. This gets passed along directly to the baby. Doctors have found a connection between autoimmune and mood disorders and babies born with yeast or fungus that has turned toxic and polluted the brain. Illnesses like depression and anxiety can take root, at their very early stages, in the womb.

Now is the time to incorporate probiotics into our diet more than ever. Traditionally, all cultures have had their own practices of eating probiotics, including injera in Africa, sauerkraut and beer in Europe, olives in Mediterranean climates, and wine in France. We've lost this practice within our modern diets. If we want radiant health, we must reestablish this practice, ideally with each meal.

How Probiotics Work

Probiotics predigest our food, which is especially helpful with harder to digest foods such as meat. This is where the tradition of a glass of wine with steak originates. In Chinese Medicine, probiotics are classified as "tonics," meaning they initiate change. They do this by:

• enhancing the immune system (which exists mostly in the gut)
• promoting regular bowel movements
• converting nutrients into absorbable compounds
• producing antioxidants
• helping with skin conditions (especially when applied topically)
• reducing cholesterol
• maintaining bone health by making minerals more absorbable (minerals in supplements are not absorbable on their own)
• maintaining a good mood and cognitive function
• removing pesticides and heavy metals from the body

This last bullet point is particularly important, as much of our modern food supply contains toxins we may not be aware of. Mercury, for example, is a brain toxin. "The UltraMind Solution: Fix Your Broken Brain by Healing Your Body First" by Dr. Mark Hyman connects declining brain power to the toxins in our system. We can get mercury poisoning from eating too much big fish like tuna (smaller fish contain fewer toxins and usually come from safer water sources). Fortunately, we can help our body's natural detoxification process along with probiotics and education as to which foods heal and harm.

Jordan Rubin, the founder of Garden of Life, is another contemporary researcher who has realized exactly how powerful probiotics are. He was able to cure his Crohn's disease, typically considered "chronic," through whole foods and probiotics.

Dr. Natasha Campbell-McBride is yet another example. She found that all children with brain disorders also had digestive problems, and so did their mothers. She was able to treat her son's autism with what she called the GAPS diet (Gut And Psychology Syndrome), which is a combination of probiotics and saturated fat.

(As an important side note, I'm not of the traditional western mindset wherein autism necessarily *needs* "curing." Many other cultures outside our own view neurological differences as gifts. It is our consumer mindset that views people on the spectrum in terms of their ability to function within our capitalist society. In other cultures, "high functioning" might not mean having the ability to work a 9-5 but rather the ability to, say, communicate with plants or reach higher levels of consciousness, which someone classified as "low-functioning" might be extremely capable of. Perhaps we can view certain "abnormalities" as special gifts, even guardian angels, rather than setbacks, through which the individual can see things that many others cannot. In this way, they play a special role in healing and elevating our society when offered the chance and given support.)

Where Can We Find Probiotics?

The simplest way for many of us to get our probiotics is through supplements. Garden of Life has a line called Primal Defense that is available at Whole Foods. It's great quality, though a little pricey. I recommend this brand to those who have been sick or are recovering from an illness. As I've mentioned, the founder of the company cured his Crohn's Disease, a disease of the intestinal tract, with probiotic dirt. Alternatively, Jarodophilus is very good and easier on the budget. Dr. Ohhira's probiotics are vegan and can be purchased at drohhiraprobiotics.com. As a general rule, look for probiotics that contain at least six different strains of bacteria. The downside to supplements, though, is they can be killed if stomach acid is too high. The best way to boost ourselves with probiotics that will synergistically work with our bodies is to eat and drink them.

Try kombucha, a fermented sweet tea. It's also great for the liver and detoxi-fying. It detoxifies because of its gluconic acid content. This acid is responsible for the carbonation in kombucha, and it extracts toxins from the blood and body. Kombucha also improves pancreatic function and helps with alcohol withdrawal. The beverage comes in bottles that are more than a serving size for people that are new to probiotics. If you're just starting out, try drinking no more than half a bottle per serving. Introducing probiotics to our diet for the first time can be so detoxifying that we may release toxins too quickly, causing "detox symptoms" like fogginess. Best to start slow and work our way up to that clear, energetic buzz we will love from kombucha.

For those who consume dairy, try kefir. It's a yogurt drink with more strains of bacteria than regular yogurt. Drink it on its own or blend it into smoothies. My personal go-to is coconut kefir which is vegan.

Kimchi, pickles, and saurkraut are fermented vegetables that make tasty additions to lunch or dinner.

Fruits can also be fermented. Umeboshi plums, for example, are plums fermented with bay leaves. They're incredibly alkaline. If we're having a stomach ache, half a plum provides better relief than antacids. Find them at any health food store (or make your own!). They're not cheap, but they do last a very long time. I've had the same pack of plums for two seasons already.

If you like bread, try sourdough. Bread Alone makes a whole wheat sourdough that's to die for.

There are plenty of fermented soy products, as well, like shoyu, tamari, tempeh, and miso. Be sure to buy organic, because fermented GMO soy does not provide much probiotic benefit.

Eating a variety of probiotic foods brings different strains of bacteria into our system. Each strain does something different. Some might help send messages to the brain, others might help mercury detox, while others still might help us make more B vitamins, which help make neurotransmitters. Whenever we see "stress complex" supplements in the store, they're made of B vitamins. B vitamins are water soluble, meaning if we take them in the morning, we pee them out. But with probiotic activity in our system, we will continually be making B vitamins and feeling their positive effect.

GMO OR NO?

As we begin to feel inspired to buy some new groceries, we might be asking ourselves how important it is to buy organic vs. conventional Let's dive in. Organic means the food was grown with little to no pesticides. If the food is not organic or labeled "non-gmo," then it likely contains genetically modified ingredients.

A GMO or "genetically modified organism" is a crossbreeding of foreign genes that do not naturally occur. At this point, the United States does not require GMOs to be labeled as such, but in over 60 countries around the world, GMOs are either illegal or must be labeled. On a very basic level, we might feel that there's something left to be desired when eating food designed in a lab; the food that's been growing out of the ground for the past couple million years seems just fine to me.

But way beyond that, GMOs are dangerous. "GMO Myths and Truths," co-authored by genetic engineers Dr. John Fagan and Dr. Michael Antonio and researcher Claire Robinson, explains that not only are there better ways to create a safe and sustainable agricultural system, but GMOs contain such toxic pesticides that a small amount can be enough to cause serious liver and kidney damage. In late 2013, nearly 300 scientists and legal experts affirmed that there is "No scientific consensus on GMO safety." Why is our government still allowing and promoting them in our food chain? Unlike organic plants, GMOs are patentable, which means there's money to be made.

One type of GMO is engineered to tolerate glyphosate, a chemical in the herbicide "Roundup." This chemical mimics estrogen in the human body and stimulates breast cancer cell growth. Glyphosate also destroys gut bacteria. This brings us right back to the issue of digestion. Without strong digestion, we cannot maintain a stable mood or immune system. Seventy percent of the immune system is in the gut! Furthermore, the body can't produce tryptophan without beneficial bacteria, and tryptophan is a precursor for serotonin, a neurotransmitter necessary for mood regulation.

Another category of GMO is designed to continuously produce a built-in toxic pesticide ("Bt Toxin"). Insects that attempt to eat these crops die from stomach explosions. Then we eat them. Our children, with their smaller, less mature digestive systems, eat them.

The third type of GMO is engineered to contain a certain trait. Here's the issue: scientists couple the gene they want expressed with a "transcription promoter," which has the function of waking up genes. Everyone has latent genes for certain diseases such as cancer. We don't know yet which genes will be woken up by GMOs, but we do know that we are only getting sicker.

Since their introduction, degenerative diseases have skyrocketed. Animals don't touch GMO crops on their own. If forced to, most end up with reproductive problems, high blood sugar, organ anomalies, blood diseases, or die. We are being poisoned while lobbyists make money off of ridiculous, toxic patents that serve to keep us sick and dependent on big pharmaceutical companies.

There are passionate voices on both sides of the debate. When it comes down to it, we can be certain that we don't know how GMOs will affect us over time. We don't know, for example, how giving fish-genes to carrots (to help preserve freshness) will affect us. We know what an organic carrot does to the body, but once we implant it with foreign genes, it's no longer the carrot that synergistically works within the body. We lose thousands of years of information in a very short period of time. We are right on the cusp of seeing this tragedy come to pass.

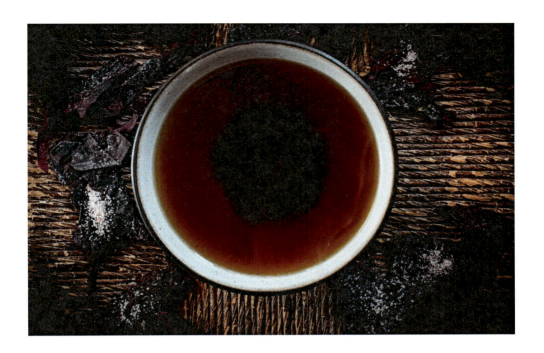

Misty Eyed Miso Soup

A simple recipe that works synergistically within the body and boasts a healthy dose of pro-biotics. This miso soup is one of the easiest-to-prepare regeneration foods on the planet.

Ingredients:

•Organic miso

•Wakame flakes

•Optional: scallions, tofu, sesame oil

1. Boil water.
2. Turn off the fire and stir in miso paste. About one heaping teaspoon per serving.
3. Add your seaweed of choice. Wakame flakes or nori strips are great here.
4. Garnish with scallions, tiny tofu chunks, and a dash of sesame oil. (optional)
5. Drink once a day for a happy gut and less bloating.

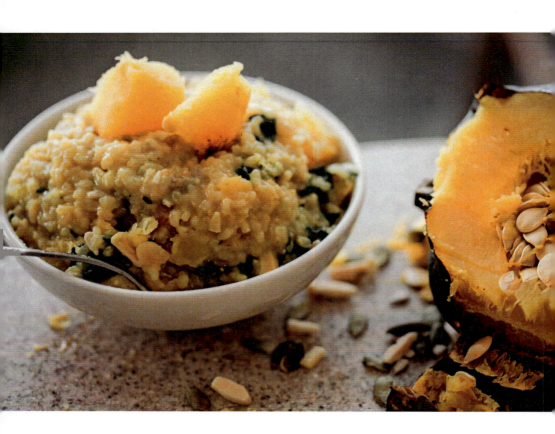

2

SMOOTH MOVES, FOR-EVER

Let's be honest: When we're constipated, toxins are circulating around the body and making us feel crappy. We should be going to the bathroom at least once a day. According to traditional Chinese medicine, we should go first thing in the morning, before breakfast, require little to no toilet paper, and create almost no smell. These are indications that things are working properly.

The good news is that constipation is entirely avoidable. *The secret formula to smooth moves is liquid + fat + fiber.*

Here's a list of foods and practices that can help:

- Water. This is number one. Liquids are our best friends when we're constipated.
- Herbal tea
- Chia seeds (soaked in aloe vera juice, coconut milk, or kefir)
- Flax seeds (ground)
- Chlorella tablets
- Aloe vera juice or gel
- Avocados
- Nuts
- Oil
- Magnesium
- Removing gluten from the diet
- Fiber from vegetables, not grains (try sunflower sprouts!)
- Avoiding painkillers
- Squatting on the toilet instead of sitting upright

The opposite of constipation is, of course, not great for our mood either. In this case, reduce your intake of cold foods and drinks and try sour foods like lemon and raw apple cider vinegar. In both cases, probiotics are helpful.

Moody Magnesium Sticky Rice

The ingredients in this tasty bowl of happiness are all great sources of magnesium, a mineral associated with mental and physical relaxation. Most Americans have a magnesium deficiency due to the depleted quality of our soil. Incorporating these simple, whole foods into my diet on a daily basis was a game changer in my digestive efforts.

Ingredients:

•2 cups brown rice

•1 can of coconut milk

•1 whole acorn squash

•1 bunch of spinach

•1 handful of almonds

•1 handful of sunflower
  seeds

•Sea salt to taste

•*For spice-lovers add*:

•¼ teaspoon chili, coriander, cumin, and turmeric

•*For the spice-averse*:

•½ teaspoon cinnamon and nutmeg

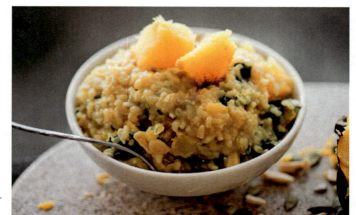

1. Rinse the rice before soaking it for at least 6 hours in water with lemon peel or lemon juice. This isn't necessary, but soaking grains increases their nutrition and digestibility. If you're soaking, strain before cooking.

2. Roast the squash at 400 degrees for 45 minutes.

3. Cook everything else, all together, stirring occasionally. It will take about 20 minutes for the food to soak up all the coconut milk and turn into a big, sticky, mushy pile of yum.

4. Chop up the squash when it's ready and toss it in. To make this even simpler, don't bother roasting the squash and just chop it up and cook it directly in the pot with everything else.

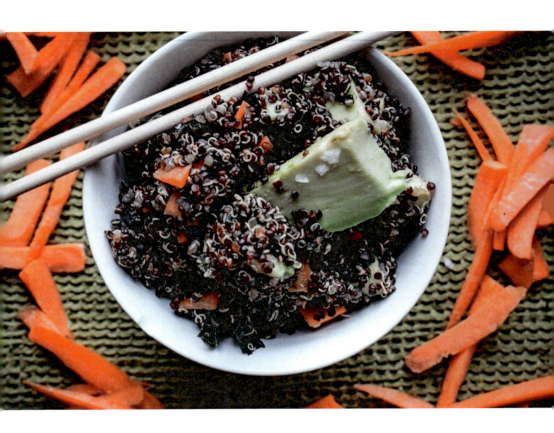

3

EATING FOR YOUR CONSTITUTION

Western nutrition promotes a food pyramid suggesting we eat food from each "food group:" grains, fruits, vegetables, dairy, protein, fats and sweets. On top of that, we're familiar with all the fad diets like high carb, low carb, high protein, low protein, foods that come out of a pre-ordered plastic case and need to be microwaved, no fat, low sugar...you get the idea. So we have a food pyramid to work with, it gets redone all the time, and then we eat the foods that make a few people very rich and a lot of people very sick.

My Chinese doctor is convinced the food pyramid is a joke. "That's a lot of food it tells you to eat!" she says. She doesn't even just mean all the servings of each group, but the fact that we're supposed to eat from each group every single day.

When I first saw her, she advised me to pick five foods that I would eat each day. She wasn't even particular about *which* five foods (I'd recommend one grain, one protein, one fruit, and two vegetables). In the morning, I should eat a little of all five. For my next meal, only four of them. Later in the day, three. For dinner, just two.

The body doesn't do as well with a ton of food all the time, which also means a ton of *different* foods all the time. We're overloading our systems on all fronts. Our bodies are asking for a break. Especially as the day goes on, the body's need for energy decreases. Our digestive fire mimics the sun's fire, because the human body is a product of evolution, just like the world around us. We have been designed in tune with our environment so that we can thrive on this planet. We are mini universes. Once the sun sets, the body transitions toward rest, and we don't need to eat as much.

The ancient system of Chinese medicine has a method to determine what each person should eat based on categories that make sense: the season, the flavor, the food's thermal energy, and the consumer's constitution and health conditions. This system has been in place for thousands of years because, when we follow these categories as criteria for balance, we actually *feel* balanced! I find this system infinitely more intuitive for maintaining good health than a system that says each person can be healthy by eating a bowl of pasta, five pieces of bread, homogenized sugar-yogurt, and a Pop-Tart. How are these allowances of our standard, government-recommended diet?

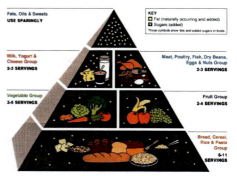

Furthermore, the foods recommended can be genetically modified. In U.S. public schools, students are taught to trust Big Agra. They learn that GMOs are safe solutions for making crops more pest-resistant and nutritious.

Rather than blindly accept the standards for health given to us by a government that doesn't prioritize our health and safety, I look to a system that promotes self-healing. Chinese medicine offers the tools we need to be our own doctors and to heal through nature's tools, without side effects and dependence.

One such tool is the notion of the "constitution." There are four main "constitutions" or categories based on body type and temperament. We're all born with a certain constitution, which is basically our bone structure. Then we develop certain conditions based on our lifestyle, emotional state, environment, diet, and genetics. For example, this book looks at the conditions of depression and anxiety and identifies its triggers and medicines. But even before we've developed our conditions, we have a basic constitution. Becoming aware of and learning to eat in line with our constitution can be very useful for finding balance and nourishing ourselves to the highest degree.

One of the first tools I use in diagnosis is determining my client's constitution. What works for one person will not necessarily work for another. This is why some people do very well with raw food diets and others feel sick and tired without cooked meals. One symptom in two different people will not always call for the same treatment. As I go into detail on the four major types, see if you can determine which category best encompasses you.

1. EXCESS YANG

This person is thicker boned, has defined muscles, thick hair, and runs on the warmer side. Excess yang has an "excess nature." They usually love rich food and have a more aggressive attitude. Without the right foods to balance its nature, excess yang may experience gastric reflux, skin conditions, hair loss, excess sweating, and high blood pressure.

This person loves steak and potatoes — foods that mimics their own intense energy. For balance, excess yang types should gravitate more toward lighter, "cooler" foods like fruits and vegetables. This type does well with raw food, a vegan diet, and juice cleanses. Fish is a better option than meat, as its thermal nature is more neutral to cooling, while meat's hot energy aggravates excess yang. If the person must eat meat, the quality should be upgraded, or they should cook more Asian style meals (think thin slivers of meat with lots of vegetables). Other aggravators of excess yang are alcohol, excess spice, and heavy, poor quality oils. Moderation is key.

2. EXCESS YIN

This person is stocky, more sensitive, has delicate or pale skin, and usually carries a little excess weight. Excess yin sweats easily, retains water, and has a slow metabolism. This is a very common constitution for modern Westerners. When undernourished, excess yin may be overweight, bloated, have swollen feet, feel lethargic (especially in the morning), and introverted or depressed.

The best foods for excess yin are warming foods that move qi (energy). This includes a wide variety of spices like ginger, garlic, basil, oregano, and chili. Diuretics like coffee and tea may be appropriate, as well, even though coffee should be avoided by the other three constitutions.

Cooking techniques that work best for this type are soups and sautés. Raw food and dairy can aggravate this type and keep it in a state of retention and stagnation. Instead, excess yin should look more to astringent foods that move stuck toxins. Some examples are pickles, radishes, and onions. Other foods to avoid are fruits, potatoes, and avocados. Yes, they're "healthy," but this type needs to limit any form of sugar, starch, and fat to maintain a balanced weight and mood. Regular exercise is another key.

3. YIN XU

The yin xu person has a fast metabolism and looks slim or wiry for most of life. Yin xu is quick, sharp, and has a knack for running on empty. This person can burn out quickly if they don't take precautions and make time for self-care.

Yin xu has weaker blood, a nervous temperament, and symptoms of dryness.

This type is the most successful with heavier foods like animal foods, thick soups, avocados, protein, coconut water, organic yogurt, bananas, and oil. If this type is vegan, they should boost their diet with superfoods and herbs.

Coffee, excess spice, and fruits tend to aggravate yin xu. Some indications that the yin xu person is not getting the nutritional love they need are hair loss, dizziness when standing up, spots in vision, twitches, insomnia, headaches, anxiety, constipation, patchy skin, and forgetfulness.

This is actually my constitution. As someone who eats low on the food chain, learning how to eat more in line with my yin xu nature made a huge impact on my mood. Before gaining this knowledge, I had been eating a lot of raw food (I worked in a raw vegan restaurant!), and when I switched my typical raw salad lunch for a steaming bowl of chickpea soup, sticky rice with veggies and tempeh, or steamed squash with quinoa, sautéed greens and almonds, I'd honestly never felt so present. My frequent migraines dissipated, and I realized how much of my natural energy I had been lacking.

4. MODERATE YANG

This lucky human has the "ideal" body type. Moderate yang is athletic with a more defined body mass and muscles. They enjoy sports, exercising, and have a moderate body weight. Moderate yang should eat a diet without extremes. All whole foods are fair game, in moderation, of course. Everything in moderation — even moderation!

The Tao of You

Hopefully you've been able to pinpoint your constitution. In case you're not so happy about yours, here's a bit of comforting Taoist medicinal philosophy:

Each of us is born with a certain "curriculum" or purpose in life, and we choose the factors in our lives that help us actualize that purpose. These factors include our parents, country of origin, and our constitution. This can be difficult to swallow, especially if we come from a challenging past. Try thinking of what you've learned from where you come from and how strong it's made you or can make you. Without feeling the victim, get clear on each and every lesson. Reframe each experience as a gift, and concentrate on that aspect of the experience. What we put our attention on, grows.

Our potential to fulfill our curriculum lies in our kidney "jing," or essence. In Chinese medicine, the kidneys are known to store all of our reproductive information or constitutional blueprint as well as our drive for life, courage, and adventure. When we constantly put stress on our kidneys, we age prematurely. When we nourish our kidneys with proper nutrition, they reward us with strong bones, good hearing, thick and lustrous hair, sound sleep, and motivation. Some foods and practices that nourish our kidneys include:

- healthy salts (sea salt, pink salt, celtic salt)
- minerals
- probiotics
- warm food and liquids
- seaweed
- beans
- pine nuts
- mulberries
- cinnamon
- self-care and cultivation

When we reach roadblocks in our lives that make us question our path and feel shock or fear, three choices arise. We can either (1) push through and keep going, (2) rear off the path, or (3) find a new way around it. Problems with the kidneys in Taoist medicine are a symptom of not walking our truth path.

Think of the kidneys as two battery packs. If they're charged, we have all the potential we need for creativity and purpose. If we don't charge them, if we lose our innate awareness of how to conserve and harness our energy, we lose the ability to transform and heal. When we honor our jing by eating for our constitution, we don't have to worry about carrying around a charger with us everywhere you go.

**Joyful Jing
Sushi Salad**

Ingredients:

•4 carrots

•1 full sheet of nori

 seaweed

•1 cups of brown quinoa

•1 avocado

For the dressing:

•1 tablespoon rice vinegar

•1 tablespoon gluten-free

 tamari

•1 teaspoon sweet miso

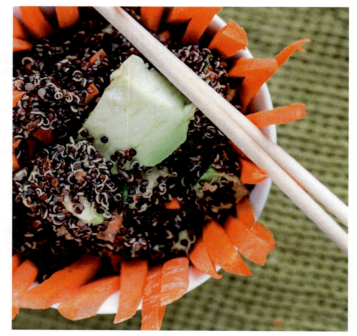

1. Cook the quinoa. 1 cup quinoa: 2 cups water. Boil, then reduce heat and simmer, covered, for 15-20 minutes until the water is absorbed.

2. Julienne the carrots or cut into small slices.

3. Cut the nori into strips if you're working with a full sheet.

4. Cut small chunks of avocado.

5. For the dressing, whisk remaining ingredients together.

6. Combine everything.

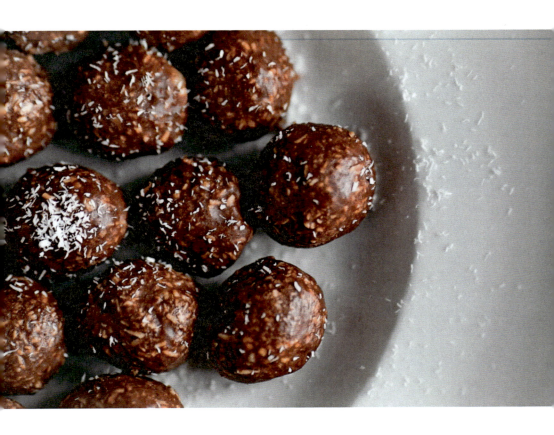

4

SUGAR SORROWS

Now that we've discovered how our digestion and constitution play vital roles in maintaining a good mood, let's look at some of the culprits that are robbing us of positive energy. When I work with clients, I ask them to fill out a food journal with what they ate, when they ate it, and how they felt after eating it. With a clearer understanding of how each food affects us, it becomes much easier to let go of low-vibe foods and replace them with better alternatives.

First, I'm looking at you: sugar, high fructose corn syrup, aspartame, agave, cane sugar, and all the many names for sugar that are sneaking into our food.

Sugar is inflammatory and feeds yeast, which causes brain fog. Refined flour, I must note, turns into sugar so quickly that the body recognizes it as sugar. When we consume sugar, our blood sugar sky-rockets. Insulin arrives to transport that sugar into our cells and our fat. As a result, we gain weight.

Sugar is addictive because its feel-good effect is so short-lived. When we're immersed in a sugar cycle, we biologically need more sugar to feel stable. This has nothing to do with willpower. Our bodies crave the serotonin released from carbohydrates.

It works like this: carbs are rich in tryptophan, the amino acid required for the production of serotonin and melatonin. Serotonin promotes relaxation and a balanced mood, while melatonin is necessary for healthy sleep cycles. The problem with low-carb diets like Atkin's, though we might lose weight on them, is that we can also become depressed on them. Without carbohydrates, we don't produce serotonin.

We need to find this serotonin balance from sweet, complex carbs like carrots, sweet potatoes, onions, whole apples, and squash. These foods curb sweet cravings and give us the serotonin we're craving.

Loaded Sweet Potato

This recipe makes a fantastic breakfast, lunch, or impressive side. I prepare the chickpeas the traditional way by soaking and sprouting them, thereby neutralizing the enzyme inhibitors that naturally cover seeds, nuts, grains and beans and reduce our absorption of important minerals and proteins, all while causing digestive discomfort! We're not vibing as high as we could be, right? We can't afford to be losing minerals over here!

The chickpeas soak overnight for 12 hours and sprout for about two days. I make a decent amount in one batch so I only have to prepare them once a week. Beans are a staple in my diet, so it's important to actually receive all of their nutrients and not feel   . bloated after eating them. That's why I make this process part of my regular food prep routine (or at least, I did before I had my son!).

The potato bakes for about 50 minutes. From start to finish, this isn't a quick meal. But, if you can incorporate this traditional cooking method into your routine, the actual amount of work in a dish like this is next to nothing. We simply let two main ingredients sit for a while, rinse them, and then combine them. You do need to plan ahead a bit if you're soaking your beans, but my other secret is that sometimes I don't plan ahead and buy already soaked and sprouted beans from the farmer's market. This is always an option if you live near a good market. And finally, if neither of these is an option, you can buy canned organic chickpeas, which are precooked. Eden makes canned chickpeas prepared with kombu or kelp, a seaweed that helps reduce the gas-producing quality of beans.

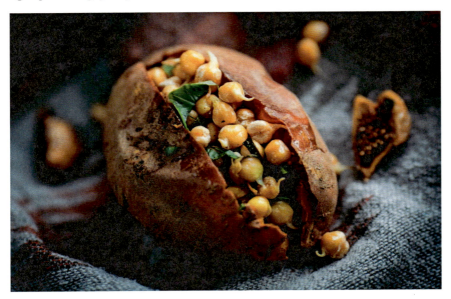

Ingredients:

- Sweet potato (serves one)
- ½ cup soaked and sprouted chickpeas
- A few fresh basil leaves
- 1 fig (dried or fresh)
- Coconut oil
- Sea salt

To prepare the beans:

1. Soak dried chickpeas for 12 hours in water. Include an acid in the soaking liquid like a teaspoon of coconut oil, raw apple cider vinegar, lemon juice, or a lemon peel.
2. Drain and rinse the beans every 8-12 hours for 12 more hours at least (meaning one more time), or 2 days max (four more times). You'll notice the chickpea tails sprouting. I sprout until the tails are ¼ inch long.
3. Drain and rinse one last time.
4. Let the chickpeas air dry or pat them dry. Store in the fridge for up to 5 days.

To prepare everything else:

1. Bake your potato for 50-60 minutes at 400 degrees until fully cooked.
2. In the meantime, lightly sauté your chickpeas in coconut oil with sea salt to taste and a few chunks of figs.
3. Turn off the fire and mix in a few chopped basil leaves.
4. Slice a slit through your potato and press down on the sides with your fingers (make sure the potato isn't too hot!), creating stuffing room for your gloriously sprouted filling.

Another way to get the benefits from complex carbohydrates is through whole grains. They pack dense nutrition, hosting B vitamins, vitamin E, magnesium, and iron. Plus, the protein to complex carbohydrate to fiber ratio in grains is spot-on. That's really want we want when it comes to sugar — attachment to fiber. Its absorption will slow down. That's why enjoying grains can be great for sustained energy and blood sugar levels. We become better able to make healthy food choices because we don't feel starving like we do when our blood sugar is low. We're even better able to exercise with that grain-fueled energy ready to burn. Exercise, of course, releases endorphins.

Many of us have issues digesting grains, and this is often because we simply don't know how to properly prepare them. When they're not prepared as our ancestors once prepared them, they can be very hard to digest, and that's when issues arise! Furthermore, for Westerners especially, grains can be problematic; historically, we've eaten more animal foods than grains. We haven't evolved to deal with them as well as, say, Asian cultures, which have always had a place for grains in their diets. We need to train our digestive systems to become grain-happy.

Here are six ways to enjoy grains in all their digestible, healthy glory:

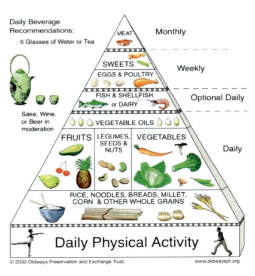

1. SOAK THEM

Grains contain phytic acid, which releases certain aromas to keep insects at bay. The trouble for humans is that phytic acid robs the body of nutrients and makes its hosts' own minerals less bioavaliable. We may be eating grains (and legumes and seeds) thinking we're being healthy, when in reality, high-phytate diets actually cause mineral deficiencies.

Nuts are high in heart-healthy fat, fiber, magnesium, copper, folic acid, protein, potassium, and vitamin E. Though they contain so much of what is necessary to sustain life, these qualities are hardly absorbable until we take care of their phytic acid.

To diminish phytic acid, soak them! The same goes for most seeds and grains. Soak your grains in water overnight or, if you don't have time, even a quick 15-minute flash-soak in hot water makes a difference. For even more health benefits, wash your grains before you soak them. Then you can actually keep your soaking water and cook with all its yummy nutrients (or feed it to your lucky plants!).

Our ancestors used to prepare high-phytate foods this way. You might even remember your grandmother soaking her beans overnight or boiling raw nuts into a fatty soup or porridge. Now we go for the foods that are quick and convenient, thinking they are not much worse than their traditional or organic counterparts. Science is catching up with the endless ways traditional foods and preparation methods are crucial in maintaining a healthy and balanced system, but the information still feels buried to me. We have trouble comprehending how our ancestors could have known the special ways to prepare food without understanding how phytates work or what they even are, but they did. They were in tune with nature and the body and the ways in which the two are designed to work. Soaking our grains and legumes with a bit of an acid like coconut oil or lemon peel (this was the traditional way) will further neutralize the phytates, as these substances mimic the acidic quality of soil. Brilliant!

2. GRIND INTO GRUEL

One billion Chinese people eat rice porridge or gruel every morning, and the Chinese people have historically enjoyed nearly the greatest longevity on the planet. This incredibly digestible food is made from 1 part grain to 10 parts water.

3. SATIATE WITH SOUP

A hearty soup is my kind of medicine, especially in the colder months and transitions between seasons. Packing our soups with veggies helps us avoid eating too much grain, and that slow-cooking helps make the grain more digestible.

4. CRACK DOWN

Cracked grains like oatmeal, couscous, and bulgur are ideal grains for the large intestine. I like to get my oats soaking overnight along with goji berries, chia seeds, and shredded coconut. In the winter, I throw it all over the fire for about five to ten minutes, and the day is off to a nourished start. In the summer, I might eat the soaked porridge without cooking it, as we have less of a need for cooked foods in the warmer seasons.

5. USE YOUR NOODLE

Noodle dishes are quick, delicious, and satisfying. Just make sure to get the highest quality noodles. Macrobiotic noodles are a safe bet. Try soba and udon. In the winter, especially, soba noodles are excellent for our kidneys and warm us right up. Rice, quinoa, lentil, and chickpea noodles are gluten-free so even easier on the stomach. Noodles should not be a complete substitute for whole grains, as they contain fewer minerals.

6. FLOUR POWER

Traditionally, bread undergoes fermentation. This is wonderful for the digestive system. Try sourdough bread, which has no added yeast, or sprouted bread, like Ezekiel. The sprouting process helps release more B vitamins from the grains.

Protein Buzz

I mentioned protein earlier in relation to grains. Too much protein puts pressure on the kidneys. Too little protein inhibits the production of dopamine. Luckily, the body's needs for protein are relatively small. Still, dopamine production matters, because it is the neurotransmitter that helps us focus (often associated with uppers and stimulants). Serotonin, in contrast, is the neurotransmitter that helps regulate our mood.

The best way to determine whether we need more serotonin or dopamine is to pay attention to how we feel after we eat carbohydrates and protein. If we eat some pumpkin, for example, and feel happy and calm, we've been craving serotonin. If we eat some eggs (from happy, pasture-raised chickens) or tempeh, and feel on-point, then dopamine's our medicine. Maybe both make us feel great. Just listen to your body. Its language is symptoms and it is a sacred communicator.

Dr. Hyman's book, which I mentioned earlier, connects amino acids, the building blocks of protein, with the ability to think straight. We don't need a ton of protein, but we do need it.

Sugar by any other Name

We now have an understanding of sugar in general, so let's take a peek at sugar "alternatives." First: aspartame. Aspartame is a neurotoxin that was introduced into our food system when Ronald Reagan came into office. Scientists who had been testing the toxin before it came into the market knew how dangerous it was. They actually had to halt their research because test subjects were becoming depressed. Diet soda, weight watchers, sugar-free gum, and so many more "diet" products contain aspartame. Gum, by the way, isn't great for digestion or gassy conditions, but if you have to have gum, choose one with xylitol. In short, aspartame is addictive and causes extreme hunger. Avoid it at all costs!

Raw honey, barley malt, grade B maple syrup, rice malt, barley malt syrup, coconut nectar, and coconut sugar are whole sweeteners. Agave is alright, but a lot of agave actually contains corn syrup. We must buy certified organic agave to be sure it does not. Also, we tend to use too much of it. It's extremely sweet, even though the glycemic index is lower than regular sugar. Having raw, organic honey or coconut sugar will do us one better. Plus, when we start to switch to whole foods and leave the processed foods behind, we stop craving extreme sweetness. Ween yourself off and then indulge a little here and there. If we can get to a place where sugar is a once-in-awhile treat, in its whole form, then we'll find our mood becomes noticeably more stable.

Chipper Chocolate Nice Cream

Nice cream has the silky smooth texture of soft serve ice cream without any dairy, refined sugar, colorings, or additives. Slice some ripe, spotty bananas and freeze them. Once frozen, blend thoroughly with a little liquid and superfood powder like barley grass, raw cacao, lacuma, or maca and a texture like sprouted almond butter, peanut butter, dates, date syrup, or coconut nectar.

Not only does this make a delicious after-dinner dessert, but it can also help ease us toward sleep, as bananas contain melatonin.

Alternatively, try nice cream for breakfast, with additions like cinnamon, nutmeg, hemp seeds and nut butter. These extras will give the body a burst of energy and get our circulation going.

Ingredients:

- 3 frozen bananas, sliced
- 1/4 cup unsweetened almond or coconut milk
- 1 tablespoon raw cacao powder
- 3 teaspoons lacuma powder
- sliced banana, coconut shreds, and cacao nibs to top

1. Blend first 4 ingredients until smooth

2. Garnish with sliced bananas, coconut shreds, and cacao nibs

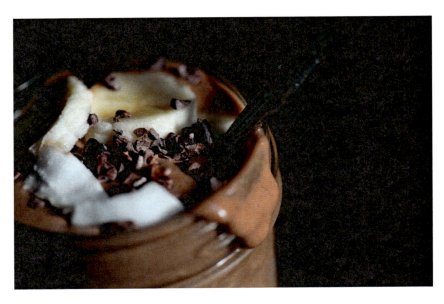

Brain Candy

The high fat content of this treat nourishes the brain. In fact, researchers have linked low-fat diets to the rise of dementia in this country.

This sweet recipe is made with coconut oil, which contains the mid-size triglycerides capable of slowing down or reversing the process of dementia.

It's traditionally sweetened with raw honey, which in Ayurvedic and Chinese medicine is known to help drive cures deeper into the body. Vegans can substitute maple syrup or coconut nectar.

Raw cacao, another key ingredient, is packed with antioxidants, magnesium, sulfur, zinc, iron, and B vitamins. It increases the availability of neurotransmitters like serotonin in the brain, making us feel happier.

Then we have gingko biloba, made from the leaves of the gingko tree. This tree is one of the oldest trees on the planet. The supplement sharpens memory and improves thinking. You can buy it in pill form and use the powder inside for this recipe, or simply buy the powder from a health food store or online.

Ingredients:

- 1 cup raw, organic coconut oil, softened
- 20 milligrams of gingko biloba
- ¼ cup (to ½ cup) raw honey
- 1 cup coconut shreds
- ¼ cup coconut flour
- ¼ cup raw, organic cacao powder

1. Mix the wet ingredients
2. Mix the dry ingredients
3. Mix all together.
4. Roll into bite-size balls and keep refrigerated. Always eat straight from the fridge as the melt in room temperature.
5. Eat two a day and pay attention to your new and improved short-term memory.

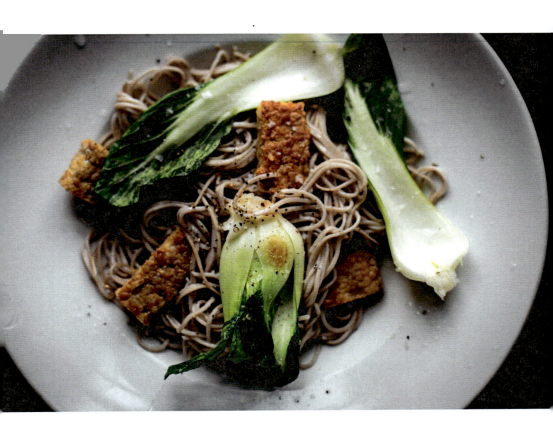

YOUR GUIDE TO GLUTEN

Gluten seems to be one of the most controversial foods today. Some think the emerging gluten-free culture is a fad. They argue that carbs *in general* are problematic, and we shouldn't victimize gluten. Some people have real gluten intolerances or allergies, and get sick when they eat it. But how about the rest of us? Can gluten actually affect our mood and lower our vibrations?

Let's start with wheat, the grain that has the highest gluten content. Plain and simple, wheat today is not what it was one-hundred years ago, or even thirty years ago! What was once a nourishing whole grain has been hybridized to the point where modern wheat doesn't even know it's wheat anymore! Originally, the government had the grain hybridized in order to increase the growth of the crop and feed more people. What resulted was a strain of wheat that contains much more gluten than its ancestor.

Gluten is a protein. It's what gives dough that stretchy, chewy, fluffiness. Most vegan and vegetarian "meats" are made with gluten (and soy protein isolate). Bread rises because gluten holds the air bubbles in place and solidifies. Gluten does something similar in the body. That's why the large amounts of gluten we're offered in today's bread is hard to break down, irritates the gut, and does not get digested properly. This results in inflammation and gas, which triggers endorphins as a protection mechanism. We get addicted to these endorphins that gluten triggers! That's why it's so hard to quit. Just *try* passing on the bread basket at a restaurant. I dare you.

You might be wondering, if gluten triggers the release of endorphins, why isn't it a "good-mood food?" It definitely does *not* make the list, because after a while of consuming gluten, the protein becomes hard to digest. This applies to everyone, not just those with a gluten intolerance. The microvilli in the small intestine begin to break, and the small intestine loses even more of its ability to digest. As

we now know, a weak digestive system makes it impossible to assimilate the nutrients we need to stay alert and happy. Furthermore, gluten inhibits the production of B vitamins, which give us energy.

Perhaps the most direct link between gluten and depression stems from the fact that gluten can block serotonin production. Cut it out, and we will feel better. If we're addicted to gluten, we probably need serotonin. It's a chicken and egg situation. Switching to other grains can help us break free.

If we can start experimenting more with our grains, particularly those that are less acid-forming than wheat such as buckwheat, millet, amaranth, and quinoa, we can strengthen our digestive systems to the point where our food allergies fade away. Gluten sensitivities are certainly real, but they're also often temporary and transformable once we strengthen our gut.

Spelt and barley are two grains which *do* contain gluten, but they're ancient, non-manipulated grains, which our bodies know how to digest. But again, if we're dealing with depression, gluten in any form won't do us any favors.

We should keep in mind that many gluten-free alternatives like bread, pastries, and pasta are not much better, because when we read the ingredients, we learn that they're refined and highly processed or made from corn and rice, which contain arsenic. Always read ingredients and look for whole, unprocessed, and pronounceable ingredients!

To strengthen the small intestine, incorporate any of these champions into your routine:

- whole grains
- seaweed
- eucommia
- siberian ginseng
- tulsi tea
- spring dragon tea
- ashwagandha

Spirited Soba

Ten-minute meal alert! This is a go-to meal for me because it's delicious and effortless.

Ingredients:

- 1 package of soba noodles
- 1-2 heads of bok choy
- 1 package of tempeh
- Coconut Oil (about 1-2 tablespoons)
- Sea salt/pepper to taste
- Sesame oil to taste

1. Cut tempeh into bite-size squares and sauté in coconut oil. Let each side of the tempeh cook for about three minutes. Add some more coconut oil to your pan as you flip. Tempeh needs a fair amount of oil to reach its full creamy-texture potential.

2. Steam the bok choy or sauté it in coconut oil for about five minutes.

3. Boil the noodles. This will also take about five minutes.

4. Add noodles, veggies, and tempeh into a big bowl and toss with sea salt, pepper, and sesame oil.

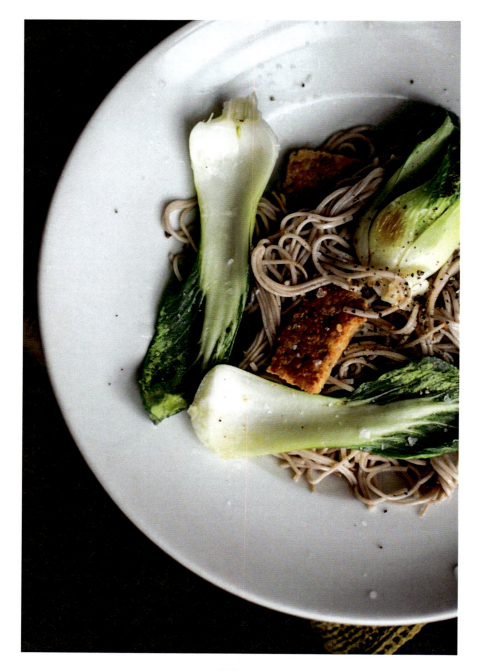

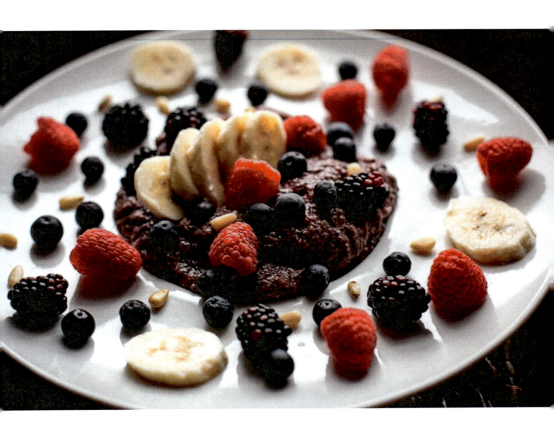

6

GOOD FAT

Another monumental issue in the standard American diet (SAD) is the mass imbalance of omega-3 and omega-6 fatty acids. Brain cells are fatty. As I've mentioned, they require a certain kind of fat to function. The brain, however, will take what it can get. When it has an excess of omega-6 fatty acids to work with, that's what it works with.

Omega-6 fatty acids do two things to the brain that affect your mood:

1. Omega-6 is an inflammatory fatty acid. When there's inflammation in the body, the brain loses its ability to function properly. Illness is inflammation.

2. Omega-6 fatty acids make cell walls more rigid, including the cell walls of the brain. As a result, neurotransmitters can't enter the brain as easily. Additionally, the placement of neurotransmitter receptors in the cells becomes distorted, blocking the reception of serotonin, dopamine, or norepinephrine. As a result, we are not as alert, energetic, motivated, attentive, or happy as we could be and are meant to be. The most common antidepressants work by changing the balance of serotonin in the brain.

Omega-3, conversely, allows for cells to *receive* neurotransmitters. They make cell walls more permeable. Receptors are not harmed by the restrictive walls and stay where they're supposed to. The average American consumes omega-6 fatty acid between fourteen and twenty-five times as much as omega-3! Ideally, the ratio should be 1:1.

Why is our Diet so Imbalanced?

First, if we're eating conventionally farmed animals, we can be sure these animals have been fed grains. Chickens have evolved to eat bugs and insects; cows have evolved to eat grass; fish, once upon a time, ate plankton. Instead, farmed animals are being filled with cheaper, government-subsidized grains, which changes the fatty acid makeup of the animals. When we eat these animals (and their byproducts like eggs and dairy) the fatty acid makeup of our own bodies change, too. Grains and corn are high in omega-6 fatty acids. Grass contains omega-3. Plankton contains omega-3.

Let's think for a moment about the fact that farmed fish are fed grain. Grain is a land plant. Not only are fish fed an unnatural diet, they're not even fed food from their own biome! We're eating foods that once contained a balance of omega-6 and omega-3. We *do* need both. Now, however, we're ridiculously unbalanced. Processed foods, additives, flavorings, colorings, and vegetable oils are pervasive. It's hard to find a restaurant that doesn't use vegetable oil. Instead of a healthy flow of mood-boosting neurotransmitters, we're left with increased estrogen levels and diseases like cancer.

While omega-6 should be consumed in moderation, our bodies adore omega-3. These fatty acids strengthen the nervous system, help fight liver disease, reduce inflammation, and, of course, improve cognitive health.

In his book "The Omega-3 Connection: The Groundbreaking Anti-

Depression Diet and Brain Program," Dr. Andrew Stoll explains the roll omega-3 fatty acids plays in mental health, especially depression. Dr. Stoll is a psychiatrist who was searching for a way to better serve bipolar patients, and ended up treating them with high doses of omega-3 through fish oil. The results were phenomenal. He also found reduced symptoms of ADD in children who were treated with the right combination of omega-3, probiotics, and detoxification. ADD often results, he discovered, from fermenting gluten in the body that sends alcohol to the brain, resulting in a foggy mind.

How to Get Back Our Balance

To restore the balance within our body, stick to fish that's wild, especially when buying salmon. Farmed salmon, although sweeter and maybe prettier, is fed a diet so out of alignment with what nature intended that distributors use a color palette to determine which shade of pink to color their salmon. This fish is so deficient that it must be colored to look appealing. Cold-water fish like sardines contain the highest amount of omega-3. Try to find them canned in water. Fish from the ocean have always been a staple in Scandinavia, where winters are dark, long, and cold. The omega-3 in fish supports their cognitive function, immune system, and fights inflammation.

More keys to omega balance include switching to grass-fed beef and grub-fed chicken and eggs (or avoiding animal products completely), snacking on walnuts, chia seeds, hemp seeds, and flax seeds, and taking supplements like chlorella, wild fish oil, krill oil, or fermented cod liver oil. Fish oil, unlike most other omega-3 sources, can be broken down into usable omega-3 fatty acids without any additional steps. The fish break down the omega-3 for you, so for some people, it's really the way to go.

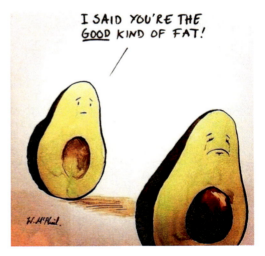

Vegetable sources are harder to assimilate. Omega-3 is broken down into EPA and DHA. EPA is the fat associated with emotional balance. DHA plays a part in the structure of membranes, which assists with thinking. If you're plant-based, you can get vegan omega-3 derived from algae. That's where the fish get it from in the first place. The only catch is they're not as high in EPA. If you're dealing with serious depression, EPA is helpful. If you just feel a little foggy-minded, DHA is all you need. Another way to maintain balance is by choosing oils that are balanced.

First: **coconut oil**. When virgin and unrefined, coconut oil is considered to have numerous medicinal properties, from helping to burn fat to improving blood cholesterol levels to helping stave off viruses. The brain needs midsize triglycerides to slow down or even reverse the process of dementia. We've seen a gradual increase in dementia in this country, likely related to low fat diets. These patients should use coconut oil. It's one of my staple oils for cooking because, in addition to its sweet and creamy flavor, it has a relatively high smoke point. This means that a normal cooking flame won't turn the oil brown, burn the food or alter its chemical properties in a harmful way.

Which brings me to the next healthy oil, **olive oil**. This Mediterranean nectar of the gods contains the perfect balance of omega-3 and omega-6 fatty acids. However, to maintain both the flavor and health benefits, olive oil is best enjoyed raw and should be extra virgin. When heated over a medium to high flame, it loses most of its health benefits.

Sesame oil, on the other hand, makes a delicious cooked dish. It has a

stronger flavor, but if you like it, it can elevate a simple stir-fry to a whole new level. What's more, in Chinese medicine it's known to be moisturizing when consumed, working its powers from the inside out. Your skin and hair might thank you for preparing Asian-inspired dishes with sesame oil, particularly in colder months when we have a tendency toward dryness.

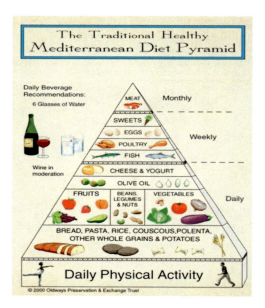

Then there's **pumpkin seed oil, flaxseed oil, walnut oil, avocado oil, truffle oil and hazelnut oil** — all fantastic options (raw only, please!). Each one packs powerful flavor and allows us to add healthy fat to our dishes. In Chinese medicine, pumpkin seed oil is said to "tonify," or increase the available energy, of our "jing," or essence. The nut-based oils work amazingly in desserts.

To be crystal clear, oil is not a "whole food." It is the isolated fat of a whole food. Though these oils are as healthy as oils come, I recommend consuming in small, medicinal doses, if at all.

Back to the Culprits

Avoid vegetable, soybean, canola, grapeseed, corn, cottonseed and sunflower oil. Each of these is disproportionately high in omega-6 fatty acids.

When we're trying to become our greatest versions, incorporating probiotics and omega-3 fatty acids into our diets is a beautiful idea. Many essential vitamins, including the "happy vitamin" Vitamin D, are fat soluble.

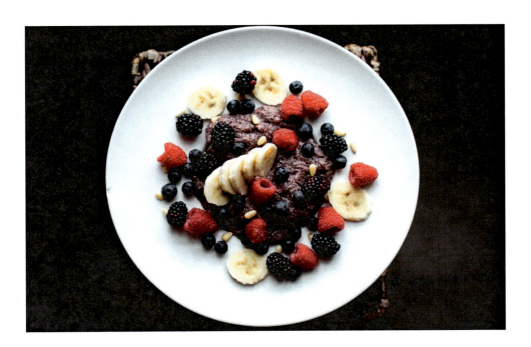

Blissful Berry Banana Chia Seed Pudding with Pine Nuts

I'm a big fan of chia pudding as a breakfast, snack, or dessert. It's so easy to prepare, and who doesn't love pudding? It's perfectly versatile, as well; you can make it your own and suit your tastes with whatever ingredients you have on hand. This recipe is for a berry chia pudding, but you could just as easily use cacao powder for a chocolate pudding, or coconut, hazelnut, or peanut butter. The sky's the limit! I only recommend sticking with the basic ratio of 1 part chia seeds:4 parts liquid.

This pudding is topped with pine nuts. Out of all the nuts, they have the nutrient content most similar to milk, giving them a nourishing and nurturing energy. Pine nuts only grow wild, so they're inherently organic and traditional, contain a broad range of nutrients, and are anti-inflammatory.

Wild foods in general offer a special energy. They grow in communities where plants are aware of each other and synergistically contain the nutrients needed in that bioregion. In South America, when shamans harvest their herbs, they begin by identifying the "grandmother" of the area through their understanding of plant growth, shapes, and colors, and then ask for permission to collect her grandchildren.

Wild foods like herbs, mushrooms, berries, seaweed, salt, spring water, nuts, honey, and royal jelly are their own class of "superfoods."

Ingredients:

- 1 ½ cups nut milk of choice (I like unsweetened coconut, almond, and hemp milk)

- ⅓ cup chia seeds

- 1 banana

- ¼ cup grade B maple syrup

- handful of berries (I used blueberries, raspberries, and blackberries)

- ¼ teaspoon sea salt

1. Blend together all ingredients minus the chia seeds. If you don't have a blender, whisk them together in a mixing bowl. Blending will give you a uniformly creamy pudding. Mixing by hand will give you some texture, which I actually like! If you want *really* smooth pudding, blend the chia seeds along with everything else.

2. Transfer the mixture to a jar and stir in the chia seeds.

3. Let it sit in the refrigerator overnight, or at least half an hour. Stir and enjoy with more fresh berries, banana slices, and pine nuts.

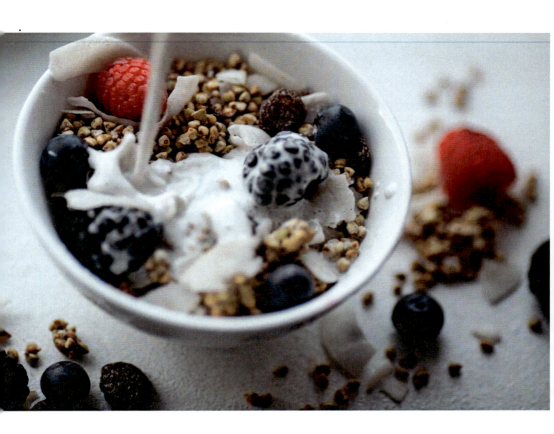

7

IS SOY HEALTHY?

Soy is another controversial food. In this chapter, we'll explore why. Soy, like other leg-umes as well as grains and nuts, contains phytic acid. We know from the chapter on grain that phytic acid robs the body of nutrients. It's an "anti-nutrient" that hinders the assimilation of calcium, magnesium, copper, iron, and zinc. Zinc is known as the intelligence mineral, because it helps with brain and nervous system function. Soaking and sprouting reduce phytic acid in all beans *except* soy.

Furthermore, soy can affect the health of our thyroid. Thyroid hormones affect metabolism, libido, and mood. Sluggish thyroid means sluggish attitude. A diet high in pesticides is one way in which thyroid function is suppressed. At least 93% of soy in the U.S. is genetically modified, meaning it's ultra contaminated by pesticides. Even if we buy organic soy, it still contains goitrogens, which depress thyroid function. Bear in mind, 96% of Americans eat a diet deficient in iodine, necessary for the production of thyroid hormones. When our iodine levels are low, soy increases the body's need for vitamin D, which as we now know, is a major player in emotional well being. In these ways, soy may not be an ideal food for a person dealing with thyroid issues or depression.

Let's also take a look at isolated soy protein, a product of the chemical process during which high heat denatures soy's fragile proteins. It's in your meatless meats, protein powder, protein bars, Clif bars, and much more. Read ingredients! Soy is an ubiquitous filler. In my early vegan days, I'd eat a lot of fake meat and dairy products to replace the foods I was used to eating. I knew they were processed, but I figured that they had to be healthier than their animal versions. Not necessarily.

Isolated soy protein or textured vegetable protein contributes to feelings of depression. It irritates the gut and can cause Irritable Bowel Syndrome. When bowels are retaliating and the gut is leaking, it's hard to vibrate high.

You might be wondering how I can love Chinese medicine so much and then say anything negative about a Chinese staple like soy. Well, the Chinese didn't actually include soy in their diet at all until...they started fermenting it! The slow and traditional process of fermentation makes soy digestible, and I guarantee the vast majority of soy you've been eating hasn't been fermented.

Fermented soy contains the highest amount of protein out of all the beans. Organic and fermented soy products are enzyme-rich, alkalizing, and delicious. Some of these foods include miso (try chickpea miso if you're allergic to soy!), tamari and shoyu (which are healthier alternatives to soy sauce), and tempeh. Tempeh can be an acquired taste, but if you're feeling adventurous, it's an amazing and versatile source of plant-based protein and a staple in my diet. One way to cook it is to pan-fry it. This method is simple and gives it a rich, almost cheesy texture. Nowadays it's available in most supermarkets. Even Trader Joe's makes an organic one.

Tofu, on the other hand, is often refined and not as nutritious. Today, it's usually made with soy fillers, which lead to estrogen issues. Tempeh, on the other hand, is made from whole soybeans, so it's a much better source of fiber than tofu. But I really do enjoy a tasty rice and tofu dish from time to time, so I just make sure to buy organic and check the ingredients for any unwanted fillers.

Happy Hazelnut Hemp Milk

The longer the shelf life, the shorter the human life!

Soy milk has become a popular alternative to cow's milk. Along with many other nut and seed milks we can buy in stores, soy milk lasts for weeks or even months. When we make our own at home, it lasts up to a week at most.

Many store brands contain carrageenan which irritates the gut, preservatives, and often sugar. If we make our own, it's amazing how much better it can taste and feel.

Hemp is a blessing here because it's already sprouted, so no need to go through the lengthy process of soaking the seed overnight before blending. This drink takes ten seconds to make, and you can store it in the fridge for a few days in a glass jar.

Try warming the mylk before using in your breakfast. The digestive system operates at a certain temperature. After fasting overnight, we should ease our bodies back into the day-time cycle of eating just as we would after any fast. Putting cold foods into the body first thing in the morning is like pouring ice water on a fire.

Also, a glass of this mylk by itself, warmed up, tastes like a white chocolate mocha (almost).

Ingredients (serves two):

- 1/2 cup raw hemp seeds

- 3 teaspoons hazelnut oil (optional)

- 1 banana (*or* 1/8 cup grade B maple syrup *or* two to four dates for sweetness)

- 2 cups water

- pinch salt

1. Blend ingredients together until the liquid is uniform.

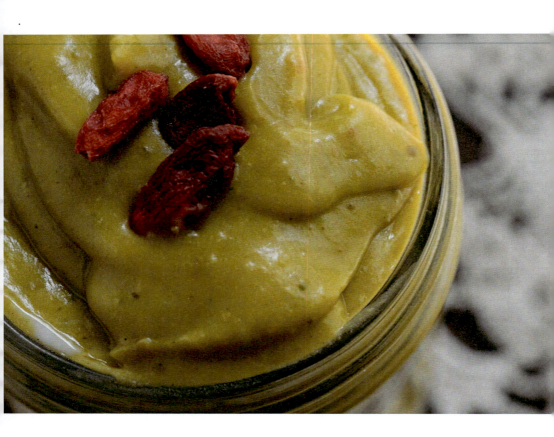

8

DAZED AND DAIRIED

In Traditional Chinese Medicine, dairy contains a few positive qualities. It's sweet, and the sweet flavor (when natural!) is thought to nourish the digestive system. Dairy is also considered moistening, which benefits dry conditions (think itchy eyes, dry skin, hair, and nails). Dairy is thought to nurture the spirit, stomach, spleen, and lungs. In the evening, it can help with insomnia. Western medicine would say it's high in vitamins A, D, and K2. Vitamin A helps with vision, vitamin D wards off depression, and K2 is linked to bone health. Sounds pretty good, right?

Well, here's the catch. These qualities apply to real dairy *only*, meaning unpasteurized, unhomogenized milk that comes out of a happy, grass-eating cow. This quality of dairy is nowhere near the quality we're consuming.

What's in Modern Dairy?

Modern dairy comes from Holstein cows. These animals are genetically modified to produce lots and lots of milk. If they're given the growth hormone rBHG, they produce three times as much milk as traditional cows. That much milk production causes inflamed udders, which many farmers suppress with antibiotics (unless otherwise stated on the packaging, conventional dairy contains antibiotics). Fifty percent of the antibiotics created in the U.S. are for livestock, because they're constantly very sick. They live with chronic teat infections because of all the hormones pumped into them in order to keep up high milk production. Those antibiotics are in our dairy, disturbing our digestion and making us so habituated to them that antibiotics are less powerful when we actually need them.

Furthermore, modern cows are fed GMO soy feed, grain, corn, and "added protein," which is waste products from other animal production operations. Plain and simple, modern cows are suffering. This depressed, distressed energy goes into every mouthful of the meat and dairy we consume.

Let's continue on the journey of our milk from cow to bottle. Once the cows have been milked, two processes occur: pasteurization and often, homogenization.

Pasteurization destroys lactase, the enzyme that breaks down lactose, as well as galactose, which breaks down casein. In other words, this process destroys two essential enzymes for our ability to actually digest dairy. Along with these enzymes, pasteurization destroys the beneficial bacteria in raw milk and breaks and denatures its proteins. Raw dairy from grass-fed cows, on the other hand, contains the probiotics that exist in rich, living soil (oh so rare today), from which the cows graze.

Then we have homogenization, the process that gives us "long life milk," the milk that doesn't need to be refrigerated. This should sound ominous enough. During homogenization, milk molecules get broken down so small that the fat molecules in milk incorporate with the protein molecules, and they gain the ability to penetrate into the walls of the digestive tract.

Now remember, our milk has lost the enzyme that digests casein. This is the reason more and more people are becoming allergic to dairy. The fat molecules also shrink to the same size as water molecules. These tiny molecules are able to enter places in the body where only water should go, and they deteriorate much more slowly. This is where we find plaque building up in the arteries. Consider this: a calf cannot survive off of homogenized milk.

It's a Calcium Issue

What's really tragic is that our milk actually leaches calcium from our bones. Doctors encourage people of all ages to drink more milk to build strong bones. But milk is not even our best source of calcium. Seaweed contains ten times as much calcium as milk. Seaweed has been a consistent part of the Asian diet, but we don't have a tradition of eating it in the West. This leaves us iodine deficient. In Western terms, an iodine deficiency inhibits cell metabolism and proper thyroid function. In Eastern terms, we're missing out on one of the best kidney enhancers, which we will dive deeper into in a bit.

Dairy actually robs us of calcium because calcium, stored largely in the bones, is an alkaline element and acid neutralizer. Milk (and all animal proteins) are acid-forming in the blood. The blood is able to maintain a neutral pH when assimilating acidic foods because of neutralizers like calcium. Calcium is pulled from the bones in order to neutralize the acidic nature of dairy. Then the calcium leaves the body through urine. The body ends up with a calcium deficit!

According to Amy Lanou Ph.D., nutrition director for the Physicians Committee for Responsible Medicine in Washington, D.C., "The countries with the highest rates of osteoporosis are the ones where people drink the most milk and have the most calcium in their diets. The connection between calcium consumption and bone health is actually very weak, and the connection between dairy consumption and bone health is almost nonexistent."

The hormones in milk have been linked to premature puberty in girls, androgynous signs in boys, lung conditions like asthma, and skin conditions like acne in teenagers. We should look critically at the standard breakfast many children eat before heading to school: processed, sugar cereal with cold, homogenized, pasteurized dairy products. This meal lowers the immune systems, increases digestive issues, and causes PMS in girls, all before getting on the school bus!

How did this happen? What happened to our probiotic-rich raw dairy?

Up until the early twentieth century in the U.S., people drank raw milk. Industrialization led to pasteurization laws in an attempt to save consumers from milk that was coming from sick cows. But nowadays, in small scale farms, where cows graze freely and eat grass, there's absolutely no reason to pasteurize the milk.

Still, this old law exists in many places, making raw dairy more difficult to obtain.

In 1978, President Carter released "Eating in America: Dietary Goals for the United States," which urged Americans to cut down on meat, salt, sugar, and dairy. The sugar and dairy associations lobbied against it and, of course, won. The food industry lobby in America is bigger than the oil lobby, just to give you some perspective on how little our government can do to protect us from Big Agra.

Seasonal Squash Custard

Kabocha squash isn't the most well-known gourd, but it's one of my favorites. It's sweeter and denser than average, making it ideal for a richly nourishing, dairy-free custard that can be enjoyed for breakfast or dessert.

Ingredients (serves 2):

- 1/2 kombocha squash

- 1/4 cup coconut milk (or more if your blender needs it)

- 2 tablespoons chia seeds

- 2 tablespoons grade B maple syrup or raw honey

- 1/4 teaspoon sea salt

- goji berries to garnish

1. Roast the squash for 50 minutes at 400 degrees. If it's organic, I leave the skin on.

2. Blend all ingredients together until smooth and custardy.

3. Top with goji berries. For the picture on the next page, I layered the custard with overnight oats (see recipe in chapter 10) for a breakfast parfait.

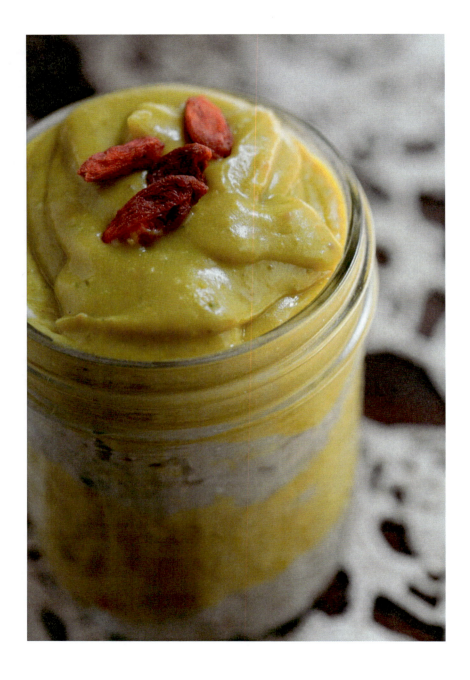

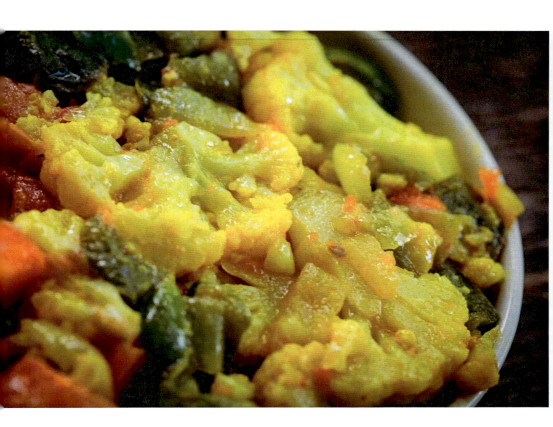

9

CAFFEINE

Ah, caffeine. At one point I was drinking four cups of coffee a day. I absolutely love coffee. Our relationship began at age eleven, when my father would offer me sips from his mug on weekend mornings. I've tried many times to give it up as an adult but never quite had the motivation until...I discovered Chinese medicine!

In traditional Chinese medicine, different foods nourish or deplete each organ system. Keep in mind that when I mention an organ as part of a TCM discussion, I'm not referring to that physical, meaty organ as described in Western medicine. In Chinese medicine, each organ is viewed as part of an extended network that functions throughout the body. Modern medicine views the liver, for example, as an individual unit that can be operated on or removed. Chinese medicine views the "liver" holistically, as part of a "whole." Rather than examining the physical liver, "oriental diagnosis" looks at a condition that is rooted in the health of the liver by examining symptoms that are visible or palpable on the surface.

These symptoms include an emotional component, as well. A bit later, we'll cover the role the liver plays in regulating our emotions, but for now I'll say that when we suffer from dryness (hair, skin, eyes, nails, etc.), insomnia, fatigue, sweating, muscle or menstrual cramps, our liver does not appreciate that caffeine buzz. These symptoms are all external manifestations of an imbalance in the liver.

Caffeine is a liver depleter and is often a root cause of these symptoms.

Caffeine in Action

It's a vicious cycle — if we're not making the neurotransmitters we need in order to feel alert, happy, focused, and relaxed, we're much more likely to turn to stimulants like coffee, alcohol, and drugs to give us those feelings. But caffeine is a short-term solution. It kicks the adrenal glands into overdrive, leaving them de-

pleted by the end of the caffeine buzz — even more depleted than before the coffee.

In Chinese medicine, organ systems are associated with different emotions. If the organs are balanced, we experience one emotion. If they're off balance, we experience another. The adrenals are right on top of our kidneys, so adrenal glands are included in the kidney organ system.

Kidneys are the oceans of the body. Oceans lie on a lower level of the planet than rivers and streams, drawing them in to form a larger body of water. Although oceans seem unlimited, they do drain off their supply. Their water can steam up toward the sky and return as rain, keeping balance between drought and flooding, or it can drain down into the Earth permanently.

Kidneys work similarly. The fluids of the human body pour into the kidneys. Once the kidneys have done their work, fluids are dispersed upwards, nourishing the other organ systems and pathways before returning, or they are drained permanently through sex organs.

Just as water is the beginning of all life, the kidneys are the source of human life. They're like two batteries that house our essence, reproductive capacity, and life purpose. They're responsible for our transformative and healing energy, potentiators for creativity, and associated with courage and willpower.

The negative emotion associated with kidney deficiency is fear, arguably the lowest vibration possible. When we experience fear, the adrenal glands are stimulated to release "flight or fight" hormones like cortisol.

Caffeine causes the adrenals to pump and triggers the release of cortisol. In small amounts, cortisol is medicine. It makes us feel awake and alert and is even anti-inflammatory. But when the fight or flight response is triggered continuously, cortisol makes us sweat and feel nervous and anxious. When the adrenals run out of energy, and they *do* run out of energy, we don't even get that focused feeling anymore. Anyone addicted to coffee knows that over time, one cup is no longer enough.

Another role of cortisol is to tell the body to put on more fat. Technically, fat is protection for the body. When cortisol is high, it's very difficult to lose weight, because the body holds onto fat for, what it believes, is protection. To make matters worse, when we gain weight, it is not just our vanity that suffers; we store toxins in our fat.

If we feel anxious all the time, our adrenal glands are overworked. Insomnia can be another result. Over time, when the adrenals fatigue, we not only feel stressed all the time, but also completely fatigued and exhausted.

Weening Off

Most of us aren't cold-turkey kind of people. If you're not one of those people, and you're looking to nix the caffeine habit for good, I recommend weaning off of it — decreasing the amount of coffee you drink each day until you're off of it completely. Switch to a caffeinated tea like green tea in the process or even after. Maybe find one day a week you can try tea instead of coffee, like a weekend when you feel less reliant on it, and then add an additional day each week.

Green tea makes a wonderful replacement for coffee because it triggers the production of theanine, the same relaxation chemical we produce during meditation. It also burns fat and tastes delicious with some alkalizing lemon juice and a teaspoon of raw or manuka honey or coconut sugar. Green tea is still caffeinated, but it doesn't spark the same cortisol spike as coffee.

Once you've trained yourself away from caffeine altogether, a whole new world of healing herbal teas will open up before your eyes. Tulsi tea, for example, lowers cortisol. It induces relaxation without interfering with focus, so it's safe to drink any time of day. It's even known to help ease afternoon sweet cravings. In Ayurveda, tulsi is used for spiritual purposes. Choose organic; tea is sprayed with heavy chemicals, and the first time we'd wash them off is when we steep them in our hot water!

If you do find yourself occasionally craving a cup of coffee, or you're in tip-top health and feel one cup a day does not harm you, be selective.

1. Go for certified organic. Coffee is one of the most chemically treated crops.

2. Buy fair trade. The source of our food matters. Taoism has the notion of "di tao" or authentic source. The energy that goes into the production of our food transfers into our bodies. Let's drink coffee that supports fair wages for farmers and workers in developing countries like Brazil, Vietnam, Colombia, Indonesia, and Mexico that work intensively to produce coffee in a system that gives them more control over their lives.

3. Look for single origin. This offers security of where our coffee is *actually* coming from.

4. Mycotoxin-free. These are the naturally occurring fungal by-products of growing coffee beans, and they make us feel even more stimulated (in a bad way!) from our java.

Avoid decaf. It undergoes heavy chemical processing linked to headaches, digestive issues, increased risk of cancer, and brain fogginess.

There are several other ways to know if our kidney system is weak. I've focused on the emotional side of kidney deficiency, of course, because that's the focus of this book. But there are other signs to look for, as well.

1. If the hair on our head has fallen out or greyed prematurely, that's often a symptom rooted in the kidneys.

2. The water phase of the body occurs at night, so when we're having trouble sleeping, that's usually a kidney issue. If the adrenal glands are overworked, then we're feeling anxious all of the time and probably not sleeping well as a result.

3. Kidney essence manifests externally in the ears. Hearing loss is another indication.

4. Lower back pain and spinal issues are also associated with kidney deficiency. The kidneys nourish bones and bone marrow; we can look at our teeth as an external manifestation of our bone health.

Aside from fear, cold temperatures and sugar harm the kidneys. In the winter, especially, make sure to wear clothes that fully cover your back and limit cold food and drinks.

Nourish the Kidneys

Now that we know what the kidneys and adrenals don't like, let's talk about what they *do* like: Minerals. Organic foods from mineral-rich soil. Vitamin C. The more nutrient-dense, the better.

Introducing: seaweed. In Chinese medicine, organs are not only associated with particular emotions but also colors, seasons, elements, and flavors. That dark color and salty flavor of seaweed gets the kidneys going. Just like in nature, concentrated minerals create salt, which is controlled in the body by the kidneys. Minerals that aren't excreted are concentrated in the blood, condensed in the bone marrow, and nourish the bones. As we now know, seaweed contains ten times the calcium as dairy, and has always been a staple in China. Unfortunately, aside from vegan and health conscious folks, it's never truly made its way into the Western diet.

If you want to try the herbal route of nourishing the kidneys, ashwaganda is a Chinese herb that replenishes and nourishes the adrenal glands. It's known to help people endure (even in the bedroom). Dr. Douillard makes a great product. Siberian ginseng is another option. Soldiers in Siberia actually take this herb for strength.

To summarize, caffeine, sugar, gluten, and stress need to hit the road if we want our adrenal power back. Take either or both herbs while recovering (and make sure to do your own research to see if they're right for you). Make a seaweed salad or a miso soup with wakame flakes. Leave the instant gratification of the Standard American Diet behind and cuddle up to the deep, lasting nourishment of the real food, longevity diet.

Anti-Inflammatory Veg Out

This dish is one of my biggest cooking secrets! The spice mix works for just about any veg dish. I happen to love cauliflower (which helps with Phase II liver detox), and the brightness of carrots and peppers appeals to me, but you can make a similar Indian-spiced dish with whatever vegetables make you happy.

This is so tasty, I eat it for breakfast sometimes! When I prepare it, I make enough to have leftovers around and I wake up craving it. If you're the kind of person who loves spice but knows it's not good for you, a little of this will give you your fix without taxing the body. It's *that* anti-inflammatory.

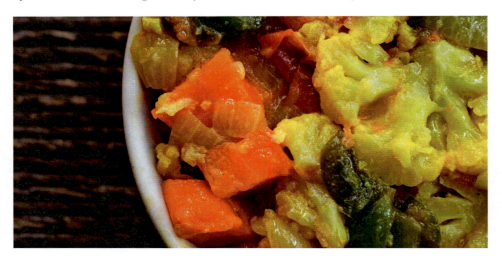

Ingredients:

- 1 head of cauliflower
- 1 tablespoon coconut oil or organic ghee
- 1 red onion, chopped
- 4 cloves garlic, chopped 1 teaspoon fresh ginger, finely chopped
- 2 carrots, sliced down the middle and then chopped into ⅓ inch pieces
- 1 red and 1 green pepper, chopped small

- salt to taste (about 1 teaspoon)
- ¼ teaspoon chili powder
- ½ teaspoon turmeric
- ¼ teaspoon cumin
- ¼ teaspoon coriander
- cilantro or dill to garnish
- lemon to squeeze for flavor

.

1. Heat oil or ghee in a deep pot on medium heat.
2. Add chopped onion, garlic, and ginger and sauté until the onions are translucent.
3. Add the rest of the vegetables.
4. Add spices and stir.
5. Lower the flame and cover the pot. Let it sit for about 10 minutes, checking once or twice to make sure the vegetables don't burn and to stir. The meal is ready once veggies are soft and tender.
6. Garnish with fresh cilantro or dill and lemon juice.

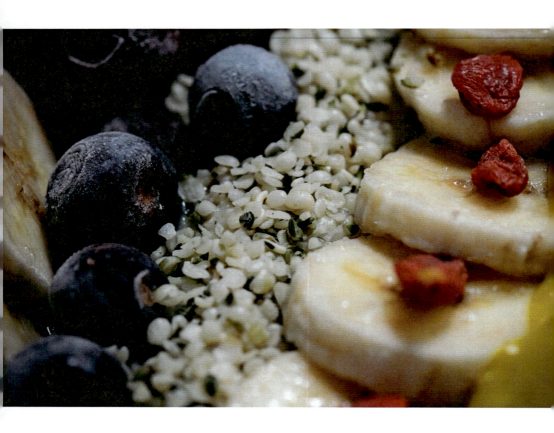

10

BAGGAGE

We've now covered the main edible offenders in our emotionally and physically balanced life. But as a holistic nutritionist, I have to shed light on a couple of other culprits. I mentioned stress in the last section. All stress, no matter the trigger, causes us to gain or retain weight, increases blood pressure and inflammation, and opens us up to anxiety and depression.We can lower stress levels through therapies like EFT, meditation, getting more sleep, herbal body oiling, and changing the situations we have control over. Let's remember that we are co-creators of our reality. The food we eat also has the power to create or reduce stress.

Gabba is the neurotransmitter that calms anxiety. The foods that produce gabba are those that contain glutamine or glutamic acid. In his book, "The Edge Effect: Achieve Total Health and Longevity with the Balanced Brain Advantage" Dr. Eric Braverman explores foods that help produce gabba: almonds, bananas, beef liver, broccoli, brown rice, halibut, lentils, and oats. We can also get gabba in supplement form. To be clear, when I recommend supplements, they're supplemental — not replacements for the whole foods that will transform your health. Think of them as an extra boost.

Overnight Oats

I eat this for breakfast at least twice a week. It's so easy and satisfying. Start with organic rolled oats and get creative with your liquid and toppings. My favorites for soaking the oats are coconut milk, coconut yogurt, hemp milk, and plain old hot water.

Ingredients:

- ½ cup organic rolled oats
- 1 tablespoon chia seeds
- 1½ cups hot water (or liquid of choice)

1. Put the ingredients in a jar, stir, and let sit overnight. Water-based oatmeal can sit out, but keep perishable liquids in the fridge.

2. In the morning, stir and add toppings. If it's water-based, I like to add a little extra hot water here so I can eat it warm.

3. Go for superfood toppings like goji berries, hemp seeds, bee pollen, cacao nibs, pumpkin seeds, and coconut shreds. In warmer seasons, look to fresh fruit like bananas and berries for topping inspiration.

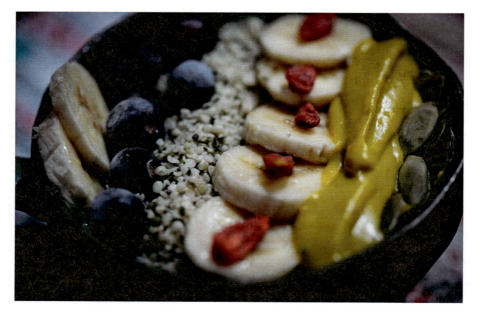

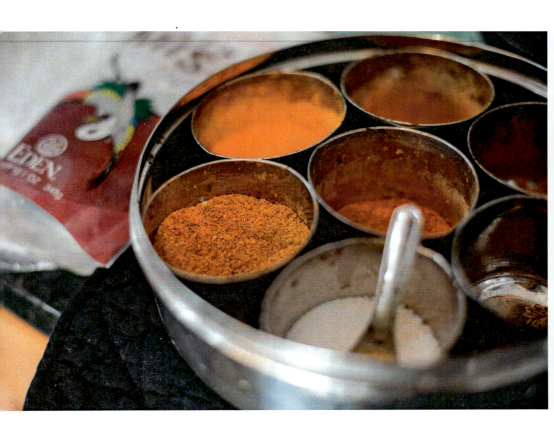

11

COSMIC CLEANSING

One way to instantly clear our mind and reset our digestion is through cleansing. According to a scientific study published by USC's Valter Longo, fasting for a minimum of three days actually "resets" part of the immune system. When we fast, our body is forced to recycle many unnecessary immune cells; when we start eating again, stem cells spring into action to replenish these recycled cells. Keep in mind, however, that this study was conducted mostly on mice, and non-supervised fasting can be dangerous, especially if we have other health conditions or a history with eating disorders.

Personally, I don't engage in full fledged fasting.

If we follow a simple, nutritious diet, our body naturally cleanses itself. But in many circumstances within our society, the body has already changed so much that natural cleansing processes are not enough to clear out all the toxins. To reset the immune system, or at least refresh it, a less severe kind of cleanse can be extremely productive.

According to Ayurvedic medicine, there are four levels of healing. The first level deals with lifestyle — diet, exercise, hygiene, and relaxation. This is ninety percent of Ayurveda, and ninety percent of lifestyle is diet.

In order to understand detoxification, we need to look at which specific toxins and organ systems we're hoping to cleanse.

Toxins include the physical, emotional, mental, and spiritual. They're all a part of Chinese medicine and play a role in why we're not experiencing our full potential for joy.

Physical toxins are often the most obvious invaders in our world. They include pesticides, GMOs, radiation, pollutants, the municipal water supply, drugs, and heavy metals. I could write books about each of these, but for the sake of this chapter, I hope it's not necessary. We know these toxins are big players in our society and that they are foreign to the body. When the body sees something it doesn't recognize, the immune system fights against it. This is inflammation — often chronic — and it's the root of all disease.

Mental toxins include overstimulation, distorted beliefs, attachments, judgements, and jealousy. Each of these toxins can play a part in serious mental illness when avoided or ignored.

Spiritual toxins stem from our ancestral baggage. Our spiritual toxins are stored in our kidney "jing" (essence). Jing includes our life lessons, karma, and ancestral past.

Then we have emotional toxins like fear, worry, and anxiety. We've talked a decent amount about these feelings already, and I'm about to introduce the Chinese medicine approach to two other emotional thieves: anger and grief.

Liver Lessons

Remember how organ systems in TCM are associated with a particular emotion? Allow me to introduce the liver. The liver, in Western medicine, processes toxins. Chinese medicine takes this a step further, believing that the liver processes and releases emotional toxins in addition to the physical ones. The liver is known as the "seat of happiness." When we are unable to release toxins, the liver holds onto anger and frustration.

On a biological level, the liver is a chemical processing and recycling factory that stores and purifies blood. TCM has found that it operates at its peak between 1 and 3 am. This is why it's so important that we're sleeping during these hours. This is the time the liver needs to successfully complete its tasks.

The organ also has the job of regulating the flow of "qi" or energy in the body. Qi regulates symptoms like bloating, headaches, PMS, poor circulation, and muscle tension. When qi is weak, the weakest organs are affected first. This condition, known as "liver qi stagnation," will often manifest in muscle tension — particularly in the neck and shoulders — as well. As I work with clients, I see that just about everyone has some level of liver qi stagnation. It is pervasive in Western society.

The liver can also have what's called a "wind" condition. Symptoms include twitching, shaking, vertigo, and convulsions. This makes sense to our Western minds, as the liver regulates the peripheral nervous system. Even excessive grooming can be a result of a fatigued liver! — think: any condition that has to do with excess movements or creates wind.

Another role our liver plays is nourishing the tendons and ligaments. Its health manifests in the eyes, so blurry eyesight or chronic degenerative conditions and dry or inflamed eyes are results of a weak liver. TCM upholds our potential to heal weak eyesight. I've yet to try to heal my eyes and forsake my contact lenses, but I believe that if I deeply cleanse my liver, it is possible.

The vitality of the liver can be seen, too, in the strength of the nails. Brittle nails that break easily indicate a need to cleanse and nourish the liver.

On a metaphysical level, the liver is responsible for arousal in women and libido in men. It holds our drive and animal instincts. It manifests as ambition, motivation, and the will to become and accomplish our dreams. On the other hand, if treated poorly, the liver will leak anger and frustration, excessive ambition, excess materialism, and rapid change. These dangers are often consequences of excess liver heat from alcohol, drugs, and toxins.

When we detox the liver, toxins get released all at once. Cleansing the liver is a powerful tool for taking back control of our happiness. So how do we do this?! Here are a few ways:

1. Water, lemon, and cayenne pepper. This drink flushes out the liver. Ideally, choose warm or hot water and use fresh squeezed lemon juice. Just a small shake of cayenne per glass is enough. Drink first thing every morning.

2. Go green. The liver loves fresh, energetic, light vegetables. Seems intuitive, right? Cool down liver heat and anger with vegetables up to your eyeballs — par-

ticularly sprouts.

3. Pickles! The flavor associated with the liver is sour. Eat probiotic-rich pickles to flush liver toxins. Vinegar counts, particularly raw apple cider vinegar. I add a teaspoon of Bragg's raw ACV to at least one glass of water a day. You can use ACV in others ways, as well, like salad dressings and baking. The combination of ACV and baking soda creates a chemical reaction that helps pastries rise, especially useful in gluten-free and raw baking.

4. Eat seasonally. The season associated with the liver is spring. The liver, along with the rest of the planet, gains an incredible capacity for regeneration during the spring. Eat with the seasons all the time for optimal balance, and in the spring, give extra care to your liver by cleansing or boosting your diet with seasonal blessings of squash, cherries, sweet potatoes, beet and dandelion greens, arugula, asparagus, mung beans, and lentils.

Autumn is another crucial season for the liver, as it prepares the organ for the good health it needs in the spring. Eat plenty of leafy greens along with seasonal liver-boosters like dill, plums, and leeks.

How amazing is nature, for she gives us exactly the foods we need to best nourish our body during each season.

5. Herbs. As a supplement to a balanced diet, Chinese medicine offers a vast array of healing herbs. Bupleurum and Dang Gui are best. You can purchase them from your local herbalist, apothecary, Chinatown, or dragonherbs.com.

With all herbal remedies, begin slowly. Some bottles recommend up to six a day, but I would recommend beginning with one in the morning and one at night, paying attention to how you feel, and going from there.

Another option is chrysanthemum, which is actually a flower that makes a delightful tea known to cool down the liver, clear the eyes (especially those that have been staring at a screen for too long), and help manage emotions. Steeping with goji berries makes an extra delicious tea and enhances the eye and liver benefits of chrysanthemum. As a bonus, goji berries contain natural melatonin. Drinking this tea an hour before bed can help us sleep better.

6. When the liver is cleansed and stronger, the ultimate goal is to wean off drugs and medications. Consult your health care practitioner if you wish to go through this process.

Laughing Lungs

As we detoxify, we want to pay attention to our lungs. While the heart in TCM houses the "shen," or spirit, and is associated with mental imbalances, the lungs are associated with chronic depression. Conversely, the lungs offer us the chance to feel optimistic and solve problems on a daily basis.

The lungs operate at their peak in autumn. In preparation for winter's cold, a stable attitude strengthens the lungs as well as the large intestine. These two organs share a similar energy of expansion and contraction. Stock up on grounding root vegetables like parsnips, turnips, and pumpkin along with leafy greens, the "lungs" of the vegetable kingdom.

The most appropriate cooking techniques during the fall are stewing, baking, and sautéing. Generally, the colder it gets, the longer food needs to be cooked. In the winter, we expend so much energy keeping ourselves warm, that feeding ourselves fully cooked, thick, well-seasoned dishes becomes extremely nourishing and digestible.

In the summer, we seek a lighter, more cooling energy to balance ourselves with nature. During these months, raw and lightly cooked foods become our healthiest choice. Our lungs love pungent foods like garlic, ginger, onions, and daikon radish. These foods contain protective and purifying qualities that give our naturally delicate lungs the boost they need.

Oriental Diagnosis

I'm especially excited to share with you one of the most helpful tools in oriental diagnosis: the TCM clock (see next page). This clock reveals when each organ system is most vulnerable and thus in great need of nourishment. It opens a window into how we can adjust our schedules to match the rhythms and needs of the body in order to live our most radiant lives.

We can also use this diagram to play detective. For example, the time of the lungs is between 3 and 5 am. Waking up during this time is often a symptom of unexpressed grief or emotion that needs to be dealt with.

Explore

Take a look at the chart on the next page and record what times of the day you usually feel certain emotions or physical issues. This may be hard to pinpoint without first looking for it throughout your day, but with extra attention, we can identify the times of day that give us the most trouble. When I started to look for it, I found that first thing in the morning, between 7 and 9 am, I would feel particularly anxious, for no apparent reason! I would wake up and go to work that way, even when I wasn't dreading work. Lo and behold, anxiety is the chief emotional symptom of stomach disharmony, and these hours represent the time of the stomach. Figuring out a few healthy breakfasts that worked best for my body was all I needed to strengthen my stomach qi. If I ever skip breakfast during this time, or I eat convenience, nutrient-poor foods like boxed cereal or bread, the anxiety returns like clockwork.

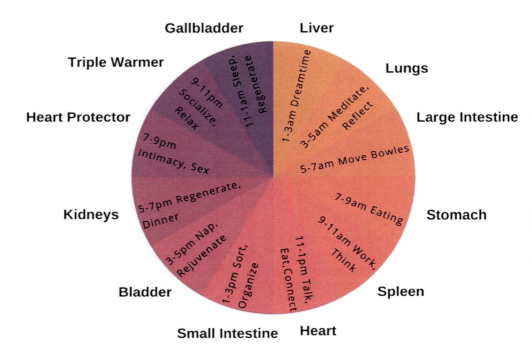

And Back to the Lungs

The lungs rule the exterior of the body, meaning both our skin and the hair on the body are influenced by the health of the lungs. Dryness or irritation on the outside is a sign of dryness on the inside. This condition can be treated with moistening food like nuts and seeds, tempeh, mushrooms, seaweed, eggs, millet, and lotus root tea.

Other physical symptoms of lung qi deficiency can include allergies, constipation (due to the lungs' connection to the large intestine), asthma, and frequent colds.

This vulnerable organ is most easily affected by invading disease, another reason why the lungs need special attention. It fits that when we're feeling depressed or grieving, we end up getting sicker.

The lungs symbolize our connection to the divine. They're the first organ to receive qi from heaven, and they do this, in part, through breath. When cleansing the lungs, finding a practice of breathing can be extremely helpful. Think about it this way: the lungs hold the rhythm of the body. To be emotionally balanced, we need to be able to control and embrace a steady rhythm.

If we're struggling to let go of grief, bad habits, toxic relationships, or suppressed emotions, it's likely that our lungs are asking for more attention.

How to Cleanse the Lungs

Autumn is the best time to cleanse the lungs through incorporating yoga, meditation, or light exercise into our daily life. Rebounding and jump-board Pilates are forms of exercise that boost the lymphatic system, which controls proper movement of fluid in the body. These are all excellent way to heal our lung qi, and, in turn, the energy flow of our minds and bodies.

As I've mentioned, the lungs rule over the skin, our surface detoxifier. We shouldn't clog pores with chemical lotions and antiperspirants that further add toxins into our bodies. The skin is the largest organ, and yes, most of the chemicals we put on it don't make it to our blood stream. But likely, some of them do. As a rule, I don't put anything on my skin that I wouldn't also put in my mouth. My favorite "lotions" are raw and unrefined coconut oil, extra virgin olive oil, herbal body oils, and jojoba oil, which is actually a wax that most closely mimics the skin and works amazingly on the face and as a makeup remover. I make deodorant from coconut oil, shea butter, baking soda, arrowroot, and essential oil. It is the best, most effective deodorant I've ever used. For sunscreen, I use red raspberry seed oil, an oil that naturally contains SPF. I mix 15 drops of raspberry oil with 2 ounces of coconut oil before applying.

Whenever we're shifting toward the more natural approach, the body may need a few days or even weeks to adjust. There is no need to be dismayed if at first you find these alternative hygiene methods less effective than what you're used to. The body becomes physically addicted to the chemicals we feed it, and the only way to break this cycle is to go through detoxification and the symptoms it may present. As long as we're aware that it isn't always the smoothest transition, we can stay strong in our decision and ultimately feel much more in control of our health for the long run.

A few other skin detoxifiers:

• Take a bath with epsom salt and baking soda. This is an especially great detox for candida.

• Use a body brush made from banana leaf fibers over your whole body, limbs to heart, before you shower or exercise. Alternatively, use gharshana gloves made from raw silk. These products absorb the static charge from our skin.

• Drink schizandra tea, brewed from a berry that is an ancient blood and skin cleanser. According to Chinese folklore, it will "calm the heart and quiet the spirit." It also clears and moistens the eyes, nourishes the liver, works as a kidney tonic, increases genital sensitivity, lowers blood pressure, enhances energy, and works as a brain tonic by strengthening memory and focus.

Legend has it that if you take schizandra for 100 days in a row, the berries give you a secret gift. If you do this, be sure to let me know on Instagram or by email what you receive! They are available at mountainroseherbs.com, one of my favorite places to buy herbs, at dragonherbs.com, which also sells schizandra tinctures, pills, and powdered tea, and many other places, as well.

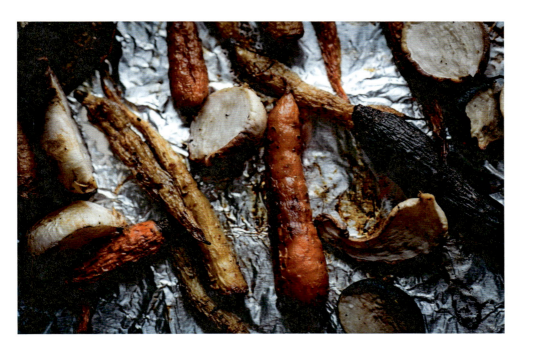

Rooted in Roasted Seasonals

There's just something about a roasted vegetable...It's the easiest thing to make and the texture is so satisfying and grounding. In this picture, I used what was available to me at the farmer's market, which was black and white radishes and purple, orange, and yellow carrots.

Ingredients:

- Root vegetables
- coconut or sesame oil to coat
- sea salt & pepper to taste

1. Wash your veggies and chop if desired.
2. Coat in coconut oil
3. Bake at 350 degrees until vegetables reach the desired texture, between 35 and 45 minutes.
4. Sprinkle on your sea salt and pepper.

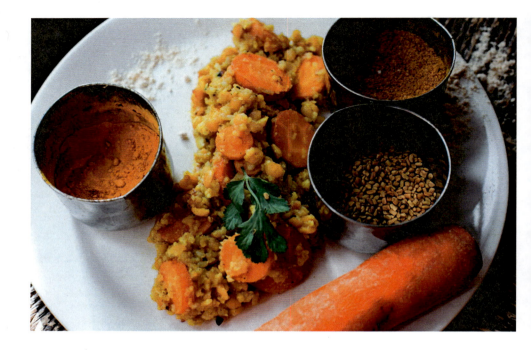

Kitchari Cleanse

This recipe comes from the Ayurvedic tradition, used for thousands of years to cleanse the body. It's basically a lightly spiced lentil stew, sometimes made with rice, that deeply nourishes.

Typically, those who detox this way eat nothing but kitchari for a full seven days. I find three days works nicely, too. In Chinese medicine, a brown rice fast is recommended. Neither of these fasts burn our digestive fire like cooling juice cleanses, nor do they leave us feeling miserable or starving.

Of course, juice cleanses do work for certain people (especially during the summer or for those who live in warmer, more arid climates), so just know that if you're not one of these people, you have options.

Take a look at your tongue. If it looks swollen, or you tend to bloat and want to lose weight, add little to no rice to the dish. If your tongue is flatter, you're at a healthy weight, and just want to reset your system, you can add rice. Traditionally, the rice and beans are added in a 1:2 ratio. This gives us just the right amount of protein and carbs to slowly discard toxins.

Ingredients:

- ½ cup basmati rice
- 1 cup split mung beans or lentils
- 1 ½ tablespoons of ghee, sesame oil, or coconut oil
- 1 pinch turmeric
- 2 pinches cumin
- 3 pinches coriander
- 3-4 cardamom pods
- 6 cups water
- 1 teaspoon sea salt
- seasonal vegetables like carrots, sweet potato, or asparagus (optional)

1. Soak the rice and beans or lentils for at least 2 hours, rinse, and drain.
2. In a large pot, sauté in oil for a few minutes.
3. Add six cups of water and sea salt. Bring to a boil.
4. If desired, add chopped vegetables. I used carrots, special liver detoxifiers, in mine.
5. Cook uncovered until the stew is soft and mushy, about 25 minutes, stirring occasionally.
6. Spice.

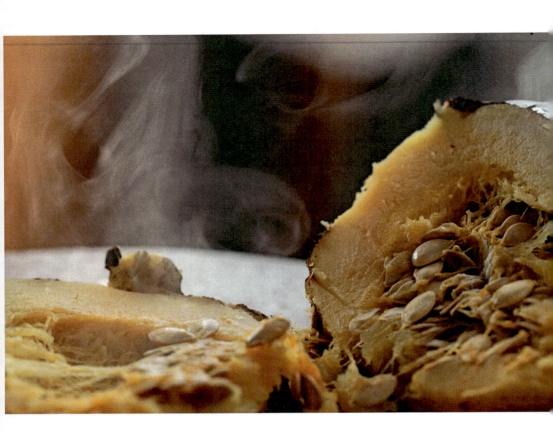

12

THE ANCIENT ART OF ALKALINE

We're going to step aside from Chinese medicine here and enter the world of modern science. Although we tend to think of depression and anxiety as diseases of the brain, the brain is not completely isolated from the body; when the body is sick, it becomes that much harder to keep a healthy mind, and when we're stuck in a negative head-space, often our physical health declines, as well. In 1931, Dr. Otto Warburg won the Nobel Prize for proving that cancer thrives in an acidic environment and can't survive in an alkaline one. Every single person with cancer has an acidic pH. But this isn't just the case with cancer. Disease in general lives in an acidic environment. To be virtually free of disease (yes, it's possible!), we need to keep the blood oxygen-rich and alkaline.

So back to Biology 101. The pH scale measures how acidic or alkaline a substance is. It ranges from 0 to 14, with 0 being the most acidic and 14 being the most alkaline or basic. A pH of 7 is neutral. All foods fall somewhere on the scale.

The human body maintains a pH ranging from 7.35 to 7.45, meaning we're all a little alkaline! When we eat alkaline foods (foods with a pH between 7 and 14), we're *strengthening* the immune system while nourishing and protecting ourselves. When we eat acid-forming foods, we're making our bodies work harder to alkalize our blood. As a result, we *lower* our immune systems and open ourselves up to inflammation.

Overtime, the inflammation becomes chronic. Doctors label our symptoms as "autoimmune" disorders because the immune system starts attacking itself. The immune system has lowered so much that it has lost the ability to recognize even whole foods, and we continue to develop more autoimmune symptoms like allergies and fatigue.

We've talked about resetting the immune system through cleansing and about boosting immunity through probiotics. Now, here's one more crucial piece to the puzzle. If we increase the amount of alkaline foods in our diets, and drastically decrease the acidic ones, we can create an environment in our bodies in which disease cannot exist! We can starve the body of sugars, alcohol, nicotine, and chemicals that keep disease warm and comfortable.

From a Chinese medicine perspective, diet is all about balance. TCM recognizes the benefits of eating alkaline foods, but also sees no issue in some acid-forming foods like high-quality, pasture-raised animal products. Any food can be medicine when eaten in the right amounts and circumstances.

I'll never forget a story that was told to me by the midwife who ran my doula training. For many years she worked in impoverished communities where the women chose to give birth at home for financial and religious reasons. She explained that a common lunch for these women was Wonder Bread with bologna. When they'd invite her to join them for lunch, she wouldn't decline saying, "I'm a vegetarian." That would make the women feel inferior. She would eat with them because, as she said, she wasn't eating meat; she was eating love. This story hit me hard, because yes, food is not all equal in terms of levels of nutrients and energy, but at the end of the day, food is how we feel about it and the energy that goes into serving and sharing it.

That being said, there is, of course, a wealth of benefits we can gain from understanding our food on a deeper level. Since learning about alkaline and acidic foods, I've cured my asthma and seasonal allergies. Of course, this was just one piece to the puzzle, as I've said. I changed my diet in many ways, slowly, over time, but alkalizing my diet and lifestyle was an important part of the process.

I've witnessed others curing their auto-immune disorders, doctors awed at how alkaline their urine is, and others who finally lose weight, improve their skin, hair, and much more. Radiant health becomes their reality!

Large corporations with a vested interest in selling acid-forming foods claim that scientifically, we'd have to eat a massive amount of acid-forming foods to actually lower the pH of our blood, so they denounce the lifestyle as myth. In a sense, they are right. What they do not consider from this reductionist mindset is that in order to maintain that slightly alkaline pH that the body needs, the immune system has to work much harder to filter out toxins and neutralize acidic foods.

Our processed convenience foods consistently stress the immune system to the point where autoimmune disorders, allergies, and cancers take root in the body. And even those who denounce an alkaline diet cannot deny that alkaline foods are some of the most nutrient-dense, detoxifying, and beneficial foods for the human body.

I'm not saying to *only* eat alkaline foods. Try out what works for you with the information that feels relevant to your life. What I am trying to say is that alkalizing foods (and alkalizing activities like meditation, exercise, breathing, and relaxing) are enemies of disease, while acid-forming ones feed the roots of disease.

I've noticed a lot of conflicting information when it comes to what is alkaline and what is not, but the basic idea is to nourish ourselves with mostly vegetables, fruits, some nuts, seeds, legumes, and a few choice whole grains. Avoid processed foods, poor quality animal products (and only eat small portions of good quality ones if you do eat animal products), cigarettes, sugar, alcohol, and caffeine.

This lifestyle is not boring! It's a blessing and an opportunity to be creative with our food. There are more resources than ever out there to help us try out some new ideas in the kitchen. There are so many talented bloggers loading us up with free, quick, and easy recipes. All we have to do is search for them online.

To simplify the acid/alkaline idea for you even more, the following is a scaled list of alkaline foods based on my research:

Highly Alkaline
Think: Intense colors
- Dark greens and deep oranges like kale, spinach, broccoli, parsley, squash, wheat grass, sweet potato, asparagus, lemons, limes, mango, watermelon, papaya, cantaloupe, grapefruit, herbal tea, all sprouts, green veggie juice, baking soda, sea salt, kiwi, cabbage, and more!
- Vinegar: Raw Apple Cider Vinegar and umeboshi vinegar. These are sthe only alkalizers.

Moderately Alkaline
Think: Grains, Seeds, Oil, Fruit
- Beets, lettuce, green beans, cucumbers, apples, citrus fruits, garlic, onions, and more!
- Berries: blueberries, strawberries, blackberries, goji berries, açaí berries, etc.
- These four grains: quinoa, buckwheat, millet, and amaranth.
- These nuts: walnuts, peeled almonds, cashews, brazil nuts (two a day maximum), cold-pressed raw almond butter, etc.
- Certain seeds: chia, hemp, flax, pumpkin, sesame.
- Extra virgin olive oil (only healthy when cold-pressed and raw. Heating olive oil changes its structure, making it carcinogenic)

Neutral to Slightly Acidic
Think: moderate amounts of legumes
- About a serving a day: chickpeas, mung beans, lentils, wild (black) rice (which isn't actually a rice but a type of bean), soy beans (all healthiest when sprouted or fermented)
- Organic raw cacao

Moderately to Very Acidic
Think: Stimulants
- Sugar
- Animal products
- Alcohol
- Caffeine
- Soy sauce
- Any form of yeast or gluten
- Granola
- Processed or canned foods
- Peanuts
- Processed or black teas
- Poor quality oil
- Soft drinks

The Grocery List

Fresh Fruits & Vegetables

The sky's the limit. Stock up on herbs, dark leafy greens, cucumbers, onions, garlic, ginger, avocados, pineapples — any of your favorites.

"Grains"

Quinoa, millet, amaranth, buckwheat. Quinoa and buckwheat are actually seeds. With these four superfoods around, you can make a gluten-free and more nutritious version of any of your favorite flour-based dishes and desserts.

Legumes

For high doses of protein, cook dried lentils, chickpeas, and black rice.

Nuts & Seeds

Try sprouted almonds, walnuts, cashews, pine nuts, and brazil nuts as well as flax, pumpkin, chia, and hemp seeds.

Nut Milk

Almond and hemp milk are my favorites. Oat milk is naturally very sweet so perfect for those with a sweet tooth who do not want to consume processed sugar.

Baking & Pastry

Stay away from refined sugar! Instead, for an angel-soft touch of sweetness, try dates, grade B maple syrup, lacuma powder, coconut butter, blackstrap molasses, barley malt syrup, coconut nectar, or coconut sugar. Don't be discouraged if you discover you don't like one of these sweeteners. Take it as an opportunity to gift it to someone you think might enjoy it and try something different. We're experimenting here! Finding the right products can take a little time and adjusting.

If you're someone who likes to bake, keep baking soda and raw apple cider vinegar on hand. These ingredients help wheat-free pastries rise. Flax seed meal works well with leavening, as well, though it offers a more savory flavor. I use flax seed meal mostly for "bread" baking (I make a loaf out of sweet potato, veggies, and flax) or in hearty smoothies.

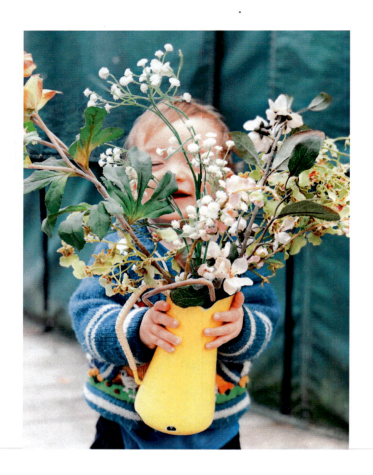

WATERING THE ROOTS

You have the tools for recovery. Now it is time to heal yourself. There's an old zen saying, "If you meet the Buddha on the road, kill him." Do not listen too closely to anyone who tells you that they will heal you. There are 84,000 kinds of consciousness in Tibetan Buddhism. Only we know how to truly heal ourselves, because no one else knows us, what we've been through, or how we're feeling as well as we do. We must contemplate our lives and figure out what's influenced us for the worse. What has influenced us negatively and held us back? How did we get ourselves in this situation in the first place? When we can take a level of responsibility and admit that we are not living with integrity, with whatever that word means to us, we begin to heal.

This can relate to any of our life choices, including what we eat and drink and the excuses we make around these decisions. You've already begun this process by being open enough to read this far. We are creatures of habit. As I stated in the introduction to this book, we consider a lifestyle or dietary change to be the most invasive form of healing. We don't want anyone to take away our cheese or soda or whatever we are habituated to. Yet the absence of these triggers is the basis of our health.

In fact, in Ayurveda, the first remedy for any health issue is hot water! Yes, just a cup of hot water, on an empty stomach and ten minutes after a meal. This simple remedy moves toxins and activates digestion and metabolism. With this, healing begins.

Remember to start simply. The cultures that the dentist Weston Price studied didn't use any technology or "science" to achieve longevity. They ate the food that was available to them in their isolated regions.

In the West, we've made diet into something incredibly complicated. We used to gain strength and power from our food, and now it's the cause of medical conditions, eating disorders, and a tremendous amount of anxiety. We can learn to eat, instead, for our conditions. We can use food as medicine to empower all stages of life.

Each one of us is a mini universe. The reason Chinese medicine categorizes each season with a particular organ system, element, emotion, flavor, and color, is because nature provides the perfect resources for us to consistently thrive throughout life's changes.

When we fall too far off balance with nature, we're left fighting against creation. It becomes us against the universe, and we're never going to win. Then, instead of living life and embracing the changes and possibilities, we're afraid (kidneys), we're frustrated (liver), we hold onto grief (lungs), we've lost our joy (heart), and we can't accept, or digest, life's possibilities (spleen). When we stop fighting against nature and invest in our health, we stop being so afraid. We can face all challenges through a clear consciousness and balanced body.

How do we know when we've found balance? We know. It's like finding our twin flame. The body and the mind cannot be separated. Every single symptom has a meaning, whether it's back pain or chronic depression. Our bodies carry these emotional symptoms as energetic charges and process them physically. So when we're anxious, we sweat or shake. When we're depressed, we feel so tired all of the time. Our bodies ache. We are in desperate need of DEEP REST. Our society is more attuned to dealing with these physical pains than our emotional ones. We casually fill prescriptions or drink coffee for energy. Rather than try to suppress our symptoms, what if we heeded them? What if we saw them as our guardian angels?

Healing is a fundamental ability of the human body. I propose we begin to see ourselves as a mini universe, grounded in wisdom, containing all of the answers and solutions within. Our potential is unlimited. Begin with a glass of hot water. This week, each morning when you rise, drink a glass of hot water. Next week, maybe make a miso soup. Skip meat one day to focus on alkaline foods. The next week, try out a new recipe. Go slowly. Be patient with yourself, and most importantly, be honest with yourself. On the other side of your worst thoughts and emotions are their opposites, so know that as you ease away from negativity, you'll be welcomed by infinite possibilities, creativity, confidence, strength, humility, and the roots of happiness.

WANT TO GO DEEPER?

I'm a certified holistic health counselor and full spectrum doula. Visit AncientRootsMama.com to sign up for my mailing list, book a 1:1 online health consultation, or discuss how I can help you through your transformation from maiden to mother. Connect with me on Instagram @ancientrootsmama.

I'm so grateful to you for taking the time to read this far and elevate the collective consciousness by healing yourself.

Yours in love, light, and longevity,

Hadas

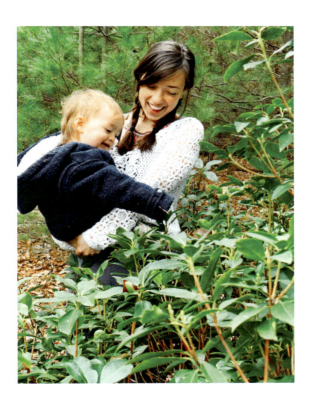

RESOURCES

Braverman, E. R. (2005). *The Edge Effect: Achieve Total Health and Longevity with the Balanced Brain Advantage*. New York: Sterling.

Carr, K. (2017, March 22). Top 5 Foods & Habits That'll Help You Sleep from Kris Carr. Retrieved from https://kriscarr.com/blog/foods-that-help-you-sleep/?utm_source=newsletter&utm_medium=email&utm_campaign=6.2.15 NL

Coffee Buying Guide. (n.d.). Retrieved from https://www.foodmatters.com/coffee-buying-guide?utm_medium=email&utm_campaign=FM NL APRIL 29 2015&utm_content=FM NL APRIL 29 2015 CID_a056b05a43c873e08b490136a3cfdd8a&utm_source=Campaign Monitor Email Marketing&utm_term=choose the healthiest blend

Dean, C. (2017). *The magnesium miracle*. New York: Ballantine Books.

Fife, B., Dr. (n.d.). Do Low-Fat Diets Cause Alzheimer's? Retrieved from http://www.faim.org/do-low-fat-diets-cause-alzheimers

Hyman, M. (2010). *The Ultramind Solution: Fix your Broken Brain by Healing your Body First*. London: Simon & Schuster.

K. (2018, June 07). How to Make Natural Homemade Deodorant | Wellness Mama. Retrieved from https://wellnessmama.com/1523/natural-deodorant/

Marin, G. (2006). Five Elements, Six Conditions: A Taoist Approach to Emotional Healing, Psychology, and Internal Alchemy. Berkeley, CA: North Atlantic Books.

Mercola, Dr. (2015, June 1). Warning: You will never poop the same way again after reading this article. Retrieved from http://articles.mercola.com/sites/articles/archive/2015/06/01/benefits-squats.aspx?e_cid=20150601Z1_DNL_art_1&utm_source=dnl&utm_medium=email&utm_content=art1&utm_campaign=20150601Z1&et_cid=DM76216&et_rid=975556768

Mercola, Dr. (2012, December 3). For Best Toilet Health: Squat or Sit? Retrieved from https://articles.mercola.com/sites/articles/archive/2012/12/03/toilet-squatting-position.aspx

Mercola, Dr. (n.d.). Study Finds Antibiotic-Resistant Bacteria Are Now Airborne. Retrieved April 14, 2015, from https://articles.mercola.com/sites/articles/archive/2015/04/14/antibiotic-resistant-bacteria-airborne.aspx?e_cid=20150414Z1_DNL_NB_art_1&utm_source=dnl&utm_medium=email&utm_content=art1&utm_campaign=20150414Z1_DNL_NB&et_cid=DM72333&et_rid=915372615

Mercola, Dr. (2010, October 22). The Truth About Saturated Fats and The Coconut Oil Benefits. Retrieved from http://articles.mercola.com/sites/articles/archive/2010/10/22/coconut-oil-and-saturated-fats-can-make-you-healthy.aspx

No Scientific Consensus on GMO Safety. (2017, December 27). Retrieved from /http://www.ensser.org/increasing-public-information/no-scientific-consensus-on-gmo-safety/

Organic Olivia. (2017, August 11). 3 Types of GMOs & Dangers Explained. Retrieved from https://www.organicolivia.com/2014/11/3-types-of-gmos-dangers-explained/

Price, W. A. (2010). Nutrition and physical degeneration: A Comparision of primitive and modern diets and their effects. Oxford: Benediction Classics.

Soy Alert! (n.d.). Retrieved from http://www.westonaprice.org/soy-alert/

Stem Cell Epigenetics: Looking Forward. (2014). Cell Stem Cell,14(6), 706-709. doi:https://doi.org/10.1016/j.stem.2014.04.014

Stoll, A. L. (2001). *The Omega-3 Connection: The Groundbreaking Anti-Depression Diet and Brain Program*. New York: Simon & Schuster.

Swanson, N. L., Leu, A., & Wallet, B. (2014). Genetically engineered crops, glyphosate and the deterioration of health in the United States of America. Journal of Organic Systems,9(2), 1-32. Retrieved from http://www.organic-systems.org/journal/92/JOS_Volume-9_Number-2_Nov_2014-Swanson-et-al.pdf

Weitzman, D. (2014, April 05). The Esoteric Meaning of Mystical Symbols & The Benefits of Sacred Geometry -. Retrieved from http://zazenlife.com/2014/04/05/esoteric-meaning-mystical-symbols-benefits-sacred-geometry/

What Every Woman Needs to Read If She Ever Wants to Have a Baby. (2015, October 09). Retrieved from http://bodyecology.com/articles/woman_needs_to_know_have_a_baby.php

What Is Wild Alaskan Salmon Good For? (n.d.). Retrieved from https://foodfacts.mercola.com/wild-alaskan-salmon.html

COPYRIGHT

Made in United States
North Haven, CT
31 July 2022

22066391R00049